PREPARING YOUR HORSE OR DONKEY FOR VETERINARY CARE

- Hélène Roche -

PREPARING YOUR HORSE OR DONKEY FOR VETERINARY CARE

Practical Training to Establish Good Behavior, Relieve Stress, and Ensure Safety

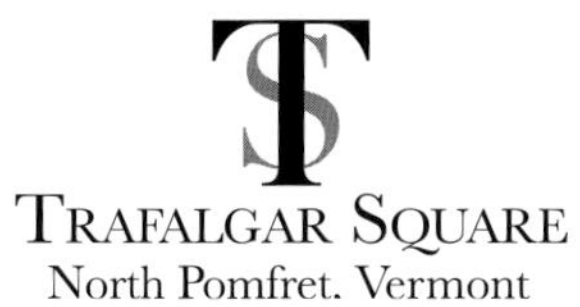

TRAFALGAR SQUARE
North Pomfret. Vermont

First published in the United States of America in 2024 by
Trafalgar Square Books
North Pomfret, Vermont

Originally published in the French language as *Préparer son cheval aux soins vétérinaires*.

DISCLAIMER OF LIABILITY
The author and publisher shall have neither liability nor responsibility to any person or entity with respect to any loss or damage caused or alleged to be caused directly or indirectly by the information contained in this book. While the book is as accurate as the author can make it, there may be errors, omissions, and inaccuracies.

Trafalgar Square Books encourages the use of approved riding helmets
in all equestrian sports and activities.

Trafalgar Square Books certifies that the content in this book was generated by a human expert on the subject, and the content was edited, fact-checked, and proofread by human publishing specialists with a lifetime of equestrian knowledge. TSB does not publish books generated by artificial intelligence (AI).

ISBN: 978-1-64601-242-8
Library of Congress Control Number: 2024933663

PHOTOGRAPHY:
Isabelle Arnon: pp. 139, 143
Alice de Boyer des Roches: pp. 8, 22, 62, 147 middle
Véronique de Saint Vaulry: pp. 61, 72, 78, 89, 141
Jérémy Durand: pp. 9, 10, 23, 57, 58, 60, 74, 75, 79, 80, 81, 82, 83, 84, 91, 92 bottom, 101, 111, 112, 113, 126 bottom, 128, 129, 134, 137, 146, 147 top, 148, 149 bottom, 157, 159 bottom, 165, 166, 167
Ludovic Fournet/Eva Garnerone/© Ethical Horse Development: pp. vi, 48, 92 top, 95, 110, 133 middle and bottom, 135 top and bottom, 146
Alain Laurioux: pp. 3, 7, 35, 37, 38, 39, 41, 42, 49, 51, 52, 151, 156, 168, 174
Anne Pasquet/© Ânes Victoires: pp. 2, 12, 17 bottom, 19, 28, 29, 33, 36, 43, 85, 93, 103, 105, 130 top, 152, 153 top and middle, 158
Hélène Roche: pp. vi, 3, 5, 13 top and bottom, 16, 17 top, 26, 30, 32, 47, 50, 53, 56, 115 bottom, 116, 117, 136, 149 top
Marie Roig-Pons: pp. 4, 27, 31, 34, 40, 45, 46, 54, 59, 63, 64, 65, 66, 67, 68, 69, 71, 76, 77, 86, 87, 88, 90, 94, 97, 98, 99, 100, 102, 104, 107, 109, 115 top, 118, 119, 120, 121, 122, 124, 126 top, 127, 130 middle, 131, 132, 133 top, 145, 150, 153 bottom, 154, 159 top, 160 top and bottom, 161, 162, 163, 164, 172

ILLUSTRATIONS:
Véronique de Saint Vaulry: pp. 15, 20, 21

The publishers apologize for any error or omission that may have appeared in these credits,
and will endeavor to correct them in future editions.

Interior layout: Patrick Leleux PAO
French editorial manager: Coralie Moutat
French editor: Angéline Plume
Cover design: RM Didier
Translation into English: Elizabeth Gray

Printed in China
10 9 8 7 6 5 4 3 2 1

TABLE OF CONTENTS

FOREWORD

"The well-being of an animal is the positive mental and physical state related to the satisfaction of the animal's physiological and behavioral needs and expectations. Well-being varies according to the animal's perception of the situation." In reading this definition, proposed by ANSES (the French equivalent of the FDA) in 2018, we start to understand the ways in which training focused on administering medical care is a factor in the well-being of all equines.

Training animals to accept medical care is at the intersection between ethology (the study of animals' cognitive and emotional capacity and behavior) and veterinary science: it rests on a foundation of cooperation from the animal to perform medical procedures, which can be unfamiliar and even unpleasant.

In preparing the animal for these experiences with care and consistency, this training allows us to make all this novelty, unpredictability, and discomfort much less difficult to navigate. For horses and related animals, it reduces fear and anxiety, and can even create positive experiences—anticipation, confidence, and happiness. It also helps improve the relationship between humans and the animals in our care.

Training animals to accept medical care is also a factor in improving their health. It makes it easier to conduct clinical examinations and take samples—both essential steps in detecting diseases and other conditions early. It also makes giving certain kinds of treatment easier, which helps make it possible for a full course of medication or injections to be successfully administered. In the case of horses and other equines, it makes owners, grooms, farriers, technicians, trainers, and, of course, veterinarians more comfortable in their work with the animal. So it's an important consideration for everyone in the equestrian world.

For all these reasons, in addition to the increased attention of society in general to issues of animal welfare, we have decided, within the French Animal Welfare Chair (Chaire Bien-Être Animal), to address this type of training. In 2021, partnering with Hélène Roche (the author of this book), I co-developed a training course dedicated to professionals, provided at an INRAE (Institut National de Recherche pour l'Agriculture, l'Alimentation, et l'Environnement—the French National Institute of Research for Agriculture,

Food, and the Environment) station. This training course aimed to illuminate the theory and methodology behind training animals to accept medical care, allowing these professionals to engage in that training in their daily work.

The goal of this book is to share the fundamentals and techniques from that training course with everyone in the equestrian world, and to make it possible to train equines to cooperate during veterinary care. Hélène Roche is clear about the need to adapt this kind of training to each individual animal—all equines have their own personal peculiarities that must be taken into account. But the underlying principles and basic techniques described here, which are applicable to all species of equines, will undoubtedly contribute to improving their welfare and making it easier and safer to work with them.

Alice de Boyer des Roches
Teacher and researcher in ethology, zootechnics, and animal welfare within the French Animal Welfare Chair (VetAgro Sup) and UMR Herbivores (INRAE VetAgro Sup)

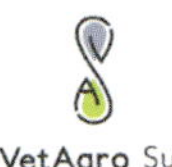
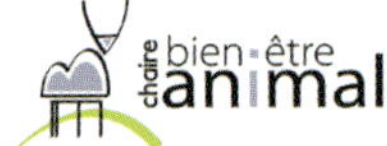

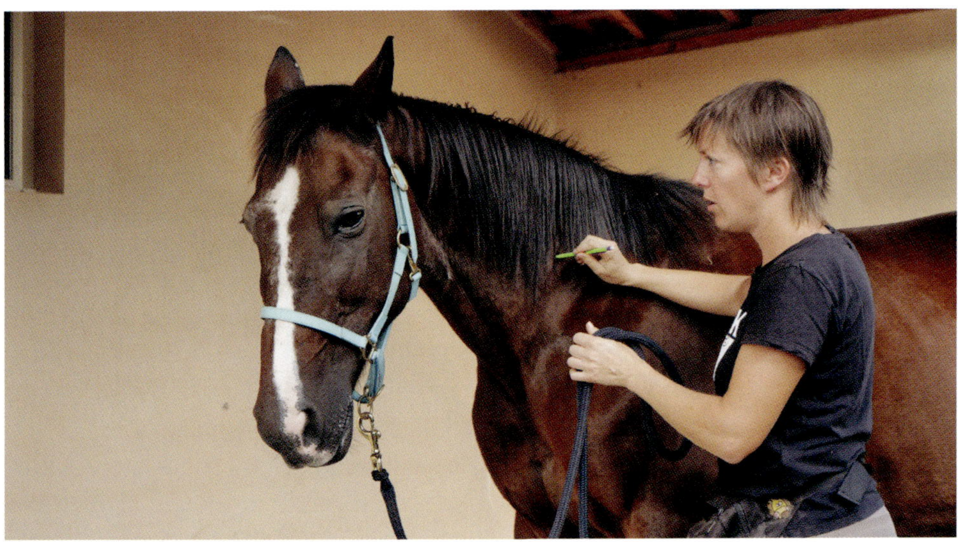

Training your horse, pony or donkey to cooperate in care should be part of your education program.

PREFACE

This book was born from the desire of horse owners, veterinarians, and veterinary students to understand how to make it easier to care for their animals.

In *Motiver son cheval : Clicker training et récompenses* [Motivating Your Horse: Clicker Training and Rewards], I described several exercises using food rewards to help prepare horses for injections, eye care, and clipping. This work was the basis for Léa Gély's veterinary doctoral thesis, "Intérêt de l'utilisation de l'entraînement aux soins 'Medical training' chez les chevaux" [Interest in the Use of Training to Prepare for Medical Care for Horses]. I had the pleasure of working with him while he was writing it, and of being part of his thesis defense in 2018. After presenting to a conference of the French National Society of Veterinary Technical Groups (Société Nationale des Groupements Techniques Vétérinaires), he won the prize for the best equine-related thesis.

Interest in this subject isn't limited to the French—the *British Equine Veterinary Association*, BEVA, launched an awareness campaign aimed at horse owners in 2018, titled "Don't Break Your Vet!" This included a series of videos showing how to train a horse to stand still while taking a dewormer, being clipped, or being given an injection.

However, since there weren't any published references or guides dedicated to training equines to cooperate with veterinary care, I put together this book as a manual, divided up into techniques for preparing for different types of care, with detailed photographs. You'll also find QR codes throughout the book, which will link you to the videos made for the "Don't Break Your Vet!" campaign. In addition, after reviewing recent research about objective pain assessment, I've included some information on how to identify signs of pain in horses, ponies, and donkeys.

I hope you'll get as much satisfaction as I have out of seeing your horse, pony, or donkey willingly and even happily cooperate with veterinary treatment—and as a bonus, this will earn you a smile from your vet, too!

INTRODUCTION

Challenges

Being responsible for a horse, pony, or donkey means providing care when there's a need due to injury or illness. Benefiting from our assistance in staying in good health is one of the advantages of domestication, for animals. Along with treatment for injuries and accidents, preventive care, including vaccination, dental care, and deworming, is also important. But no matter how good our intentions are, they aren't necessarily going to seem that way to the individual who's the most important to the process: the horse, pony, or donkey. Depending on the stage of care when it occurs, not having his cooperation can have all kinds of consequences:

- It prevents accurate diagnosis because it makes it impossible for him to be examined correctly.

- It makes it difficult or impossible for him to receive treatment because the prescribed treatment can't be administered.

- It jeopardizes everyone's safety—both his own safety, and the safety of the people around him when his fight-or-flight response kicks in.*

In order to control defensive behaviors and treat animals who are too stressed or frightened to cooperate with them, people use a variety of different types of restraints. Physical restraints run the gamut from the familiar and the straightforward—the halter, or a hand gripping a fold of the animal's skin—to the increasingly restrictive: a halter with a lip chain or a more severe bit than usual, or a stock. A twitch is one of the methods commonly used by veterinarians, but it's also a common cause of accidents, because many horses, ponies, and donkeys react unpredictably to it. Methods of physical restraint for animals are taught to veterinarians[1] because they are too often necessary for the sake of the veterinarian's safety.

---

* A study published in 2020 (Pearson *et al.*) reported that 81% of equine veterinarians in Great Britain (136 out of 168) have had injuries or accidents occur while treating horses within the last five years.

But it's entirely possible to reduce the degree of restraint needed and to train a horse, pony, or donkey to calmly accept being restrained—it's much easier to manage treatments, especially treatments that need to be repeated more than once, when an animal is comfortable standing in restraints. Repeatedly restraining an animal that hasn't been trained to understand that there is no reason to fear what's happening usually only causes a more intense defensive reaction each time.

Chemical restraints are another method some veterinarians have adopted. Depending on the prescription involved, tranquilizers and sedatives can be administered orally in advance of a vet appointment with minimal danger, as long as the dosage instructions are followed carefully. However, their effectiveness can vary depending on the individual animal. Intravenous sedation should only be done by a veterinarian, and is only advisable with animals that will accept being injected in the first place.

Having the cooperation of the animal makes everything easier, but this is inevitably going to be rare if the animal hasn't been prepared for the experience of veterinary care, or if he's put in extremely restrictive restraints from the start. Teaching him what kind of behavior we want from him while he's being cared for is an option that's too often overlooked, and far less common than it

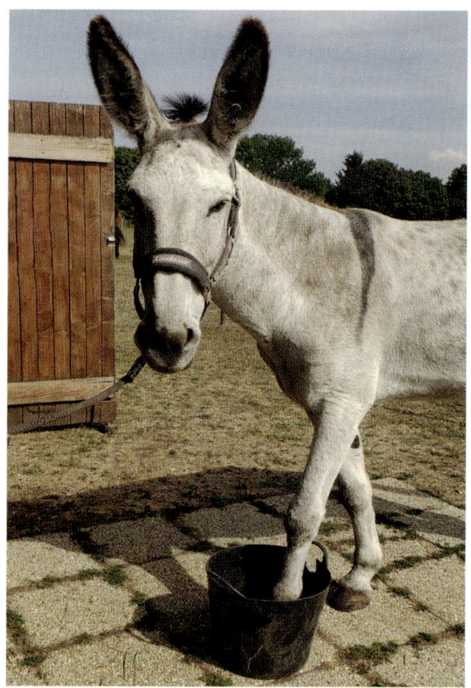

Treating a foot abscess—soaking it in a bucket like this is only possible because this donkey is cooperating with his treatment!

should be.[2] Using training, it's possible to avoid many of the problems and pitfalls mentioned above—sometimes in just a few minutes. The point isn't to stop using physical or chemical restraint at all; it's to make it possible to use them reasonably, minimally, and with as little risk as possible of causing defensive reactions with restraints like a twitch or an ear grip.

Principles for Building a Relationship

When you repeat patterns of interaction that are unpleasant for the other participant, that has consequences

Never Too Old to Be Trained to Cooperate with Care

Many people have asked me whether their horse, pony, or donkey is too old to be trained to cooperate with care, and whether it's too late to work on this with a retired horse. Based on my own experience, I say it's never too late to explain to a horse what is expected of him, and to create a positive association for him. Of all the examples I can recall, the one that always comes to mind is a horse named Sanson—I began training him when he was 24 years old. "Training" is a word that encompasses so much; I took the time to build a positive relationship with him.

He'd been one of many horses in a riding club, from the age of 3 to the age of 18, and he reacted violently to attempts to provide medical care or even put a blanket on him. He lived in the meadow next to a horse I was boarding at the same club, and since no one could catch him anymore, he hadn't been dewormed or vaccinated and hadn't had his hooves trimmed for a full year before I looked into his case. I practiced approach-and-retreat with him until he let me touch him, and then I gave him a reward and a scratch. After that, I put a halter on him and then fed him every day for the next ten days. Then I was able to get him to cooperate with deworming with a relaxed lead line. He backed away at first, when he saw the deworming syringe in my hand, but I used approach-and-retreat again to let him get used to the unfamiliar object, and the clicker training work I had already taught him. It didn't take long before he let me come toward him with the syringe. The other care he needed didn't pose a problem as long as I signaled to him with a click of my tongue first and gave him a reward afterward. I kept taking care of him, and we became friends. In the last few weeks of his life, at age 27, a friend and I had to apply medication to his eyes—and we did it without any problems, with Sanson at liberty in his meadow.

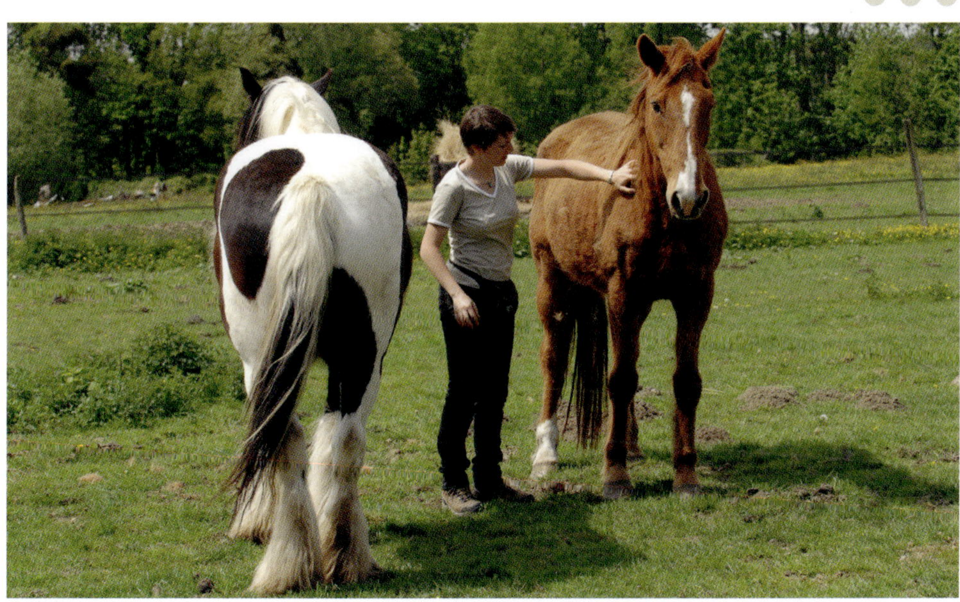

Sanson in the "re-taming" phase, at the age of 24. Within a few days, he learned to cooperate with veterinary care, even though he had a reputation for being difficult to handle.

for your relationship with them—as true with equines as it is with any other living thing.

As Robert Hinde, a British zoologist and ethologist, put it,[3] a relationship is the sum of a set of interactions. Each interaction has a tone, a mood, that will influence the tone and mood of the next interaction. So we have a good reason to try to make an animal feel good about any and every interaction we have with him.

It's not a secret that veterinary care makes that task harder—many animals, equines included, find it stressful and frightening. But we are luckier than our animals: we know this, and we're able to understand why it's happening. We can anticipate that veterinary care might pose a problem, and we can prepare for it and make an effort to counteract any discomfort with positive experiences.[4]

Tigers Are Easier to Administer Care to than Ponies

Having an animal cooperate with his own veterinary care isn't just a nice fantasy. You might already know that it's possible with wild animals in parks and zoos—for example, there's a video that was filmed at the Copenhagen Zoo of a tiger positioning himself so that his trainer can take a blood sample from his tail, and waiting patiently through the procedure until it's complete.[5]

When we struggle with a pet cat who turns into a clawing, hissing bar of soap slipping out of our hands at every turn during a simple checkup at the vet, seeing this kind of cooperation in a wild predator leaves us scratching our heads—which explains the 45 million views that the Copenhagen Zoo video has on YouTube!

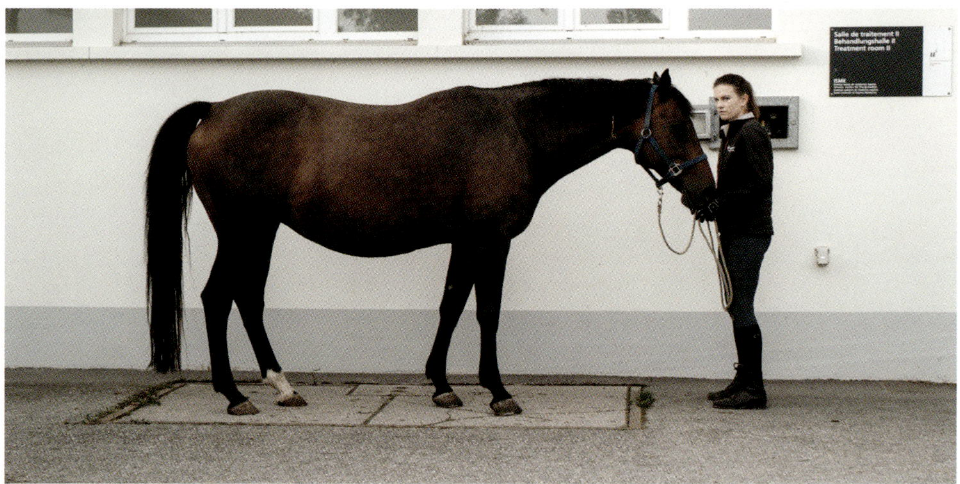

You have in your hands a lead rope, a halter, and a domestic animal. This is all you need—just remember that it's possible to weigh a wild okapi without any additional restraints, if the animal's been trained using rewards!

Behind a masterful demonstration like that of the tiger trainer from the Copenhagen Zoo, there are many hours of hard work and very advanced know-how. But there's good news: this know-how can be yours. With systematic training for humans, felines, and equines alike, veterinary care doesn't need to be an ordeal for anyone.

It might seem strange to you that wild animals who are living in captivity are better trained to cooperate with care than domestic pets, and that knowledge of how to train animals like this isn't more common. To explain this counterintuitive state of affairs, we have to look back at the history of training animals to receive veterinary care—also called *medical training.* I've been observing this field for 20 years (2000–2020) in the horse world in France, and in the world of clicker training in both France and the US. In the 1960s and 1970s, cetaceans—dolphins of various species and orca whales—were presented in captivity in water parks, especially in the US.[6]

Research on the learning abilities of animals took off at around the same time. The studies of the American researcher Burrhus Frederic Skinner (1904–1990) were widely publicized, enough so that both the US Army and American water park managers began to take an interest in them. Some people, like behavioral psychologist and marine mammal biologist Karen Pryor,[7] transferred the principles of "learning theories" developed by studying rats, pigeons, dogs, and cats to various marine mammals living in captivity. They had more than one reason to try it: not only would shows be more interesting if the animals were able to do more than just swim in a circle in a pool, but it would be easier to study them, and easier to care for them. Training cetaceans to cooperate was a particularly promising avenue to explore because marine mammals have no involuntary breathing reflex; sedating them prevents them from breathing on their own, which means they need a respirator to survive it.

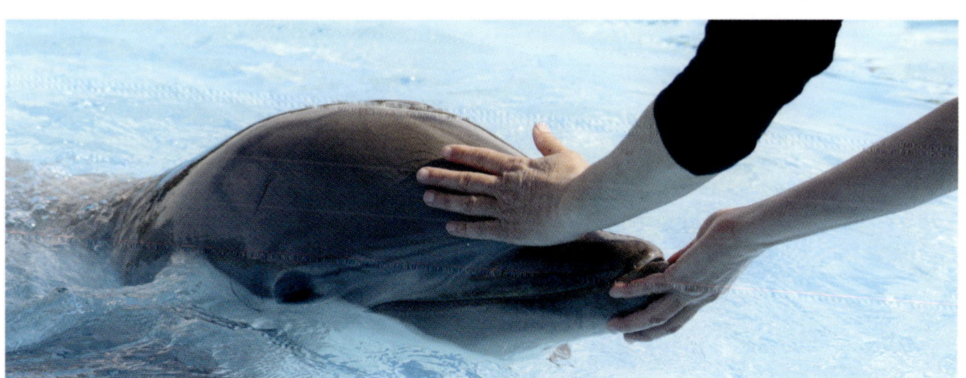

Training animals to cooperate with veterinary care is particularly common in zoos, and particularly for cetaceans, who can't be sedated without a species-specific respirator.

Complicating matters even further, aquatic environments also make physical restraint more difficult. Nets intended to trap animals and hold them still both frighten them and risk injuring them. The pioneers who tried to figure out how to communicate with marine mammals used the work of Skinner and his doctoral students, and applied it in the pool. Little by little, they managed to obtain specific behaviors on request, and then developed more advanced techniques of their own—including *clicker training*. This way of administering care, and, above all, preparing the animals for it, became widespread in water parks and then expanded to semi-aquatic species (sea lions, seals, walruses) and then terrestrial animals, in parks which housed multiple types of species. Many of these animals live for multiple decades; new trainers who were hired at these parks learned these techniques with animals who were already trained in them, which made it easier to progress and to start teaching them more new behaviors.[8] However, even though many people who work with animals professionally also have pets, it seems like the divide between the professional and the personal has kept this approach from becoming common with domestic animals.[9] And professionals who work with dogs and cats—and horses—usually haven't worked at zoos or water parks first, which means they often haven't been exposed to this training approach.

The techniques they're familiar with were developed in the context of domesticated animals, oriented around obedience and maximizing usefulness instead of cooperation or understanding. In the horse world, training is for the arena or the field, work or performance; administering care is the responsibility of the farrier, groom, or vet, and is only rarely considered a facet of training. But our knowledge in this area is evolving, and our view of animals is changing. Our desire to make ourselves better understood by them and to improve their well-being has made us search out new avenues of communication, and modern media—like YouTube videos from zoos in Copenhagen—has made it easier for us to learn about methods we might not have known existed otherwise. We can see the connections between the rats in Skinner's laboratory, a tiger in a zoo, and our horses, ponies, and donkeys.

A Little Bit of Theory

The discoveries of Skinner and his contemporaries show that animals are capable of associating their behaviors with consequences. It's possible to use those associations to motivate them to offer a desired behavior more than once, until they are able to perform it whenever it's requested of them. This is the principle of operant conditioning. A system of reinforcers encourages an animal to repeat a behavior, either to avoid

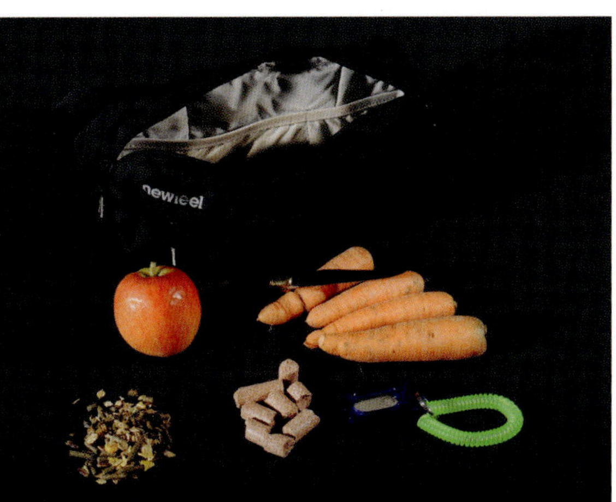

Clicker training requires rewards that come in small pieces, which can ideally be placed in a bag along with the *clicker*—but that's not essential. Another sound can replace the clicker.

an unpleasant sensation or to receive a reward he wants. Reinforcers that are perceived by the animal as unpleasant are classified as "negative," and you can think of them in terms of mathematical symbols, subtraction or the minus sign: as soon as an animal offers the behavior you want, a negative reinforcer is *removed*—subtracted.

For example, I might apply pressure to my horse's flank to ask him to move away from me. He doesn't enjoy feeling that pressure very much, so he will shift away from it; as soon as he's taken a step in the right direction, I'll take that pressure away to let him know he did the right thing. I can then repeat that pressure to ask him to move some more, until he takes the number of steps I'm requesting from him. He understands that if he moves his feet, that annoying sensation will stop.

Reinforcers that are perceived as pleasant are described as "positive," and again, you can picture a plus sign: these need to be added into the situation. If I want to use a positive reinforcer, then when my horse moves his feet, I will give him a food reward. He'll be motivated to move his feet some more in order to get more food, repeating the behavior that earned him the reward the first time.

These are the fundamental principles of operant conditioning. There are many techniques that use these principles in one form or another, either consciously and deliberately or intuitively.

The technique of *clicker training*, which I've mentioned a few times, is based on both operant conditioning and classical conditioning. In classical conditioning, a neutral stimulus (neither a negative nor a positive reinforcer) develops a meaning by being paired consistently with an event. The word "Good," or the sound of a clicker, by themselves, don't mean anything in particular to the average horse; but if, every time they occur, they are followed by the horse being given food, then an association between the two will form. As soon as the horse hears, "Good," or the sound of the clicker, he'll expect to receive food. Then the trainer requests a behavior, says, "Good," or activates the clicker at the exact moment that the horse performs the behavior, and gives the food reward again (a positive reinforcer). The word, or the sound of the clicker, functions as a marker that lets the horse know when he did what we wanted him to do. This lets the horse understand with precision what action earned him the click and the reward—receiving only the reward, without the sound or click, would help reinforce the behavior but leave him guessing as to exactly which part of what he did was correct.

When you're preparing a horse, pony, or donkey for veterinary care, it's crucial to familiarize him with lots of different stimuli.

These can be unfamiliar objects (a stethoscope, a mouth speculum, a deworming syringe), contact with lots of different parts of his body (including sensitive areas such as the eyes, gums, teats, or anus), noises (beeping from medical devices or digital thermometers, the sound of an adhesive strip peeling off a bandage), lights (for example, having them shine directly into his eyes during examination), odors (alcohol or other disinfectants, products that will be used by the vet), unfamiliar people, gestures around him, and even sometimes new places, if you have to take him to a clinic or another location. Training him to get used to these stimuli is done with desensitization techniques. There are several such techniques; all of them are aimed at reducing reactions of fear, avoidance, and flight, and encouraging calm and relaxation. Some of these techniques can be combined with each other or with

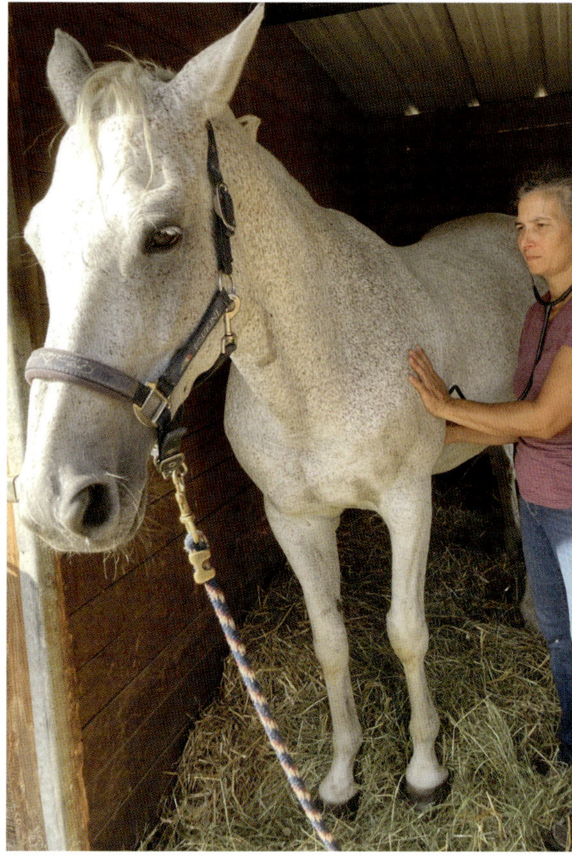

The sensations caused by and objects used by the vet may worry the horse—for example, the sudden cold feeling caused by being touched with a stethoscope.

clicker training, so you have multiple options for preparing an animal for veterinary care or intervening in an emergency situation.

In 2021, after a decade, ethology researchers reached a consensus on the most ethical way to treat horses. The International Society For Equitation Science lists 10 principles based on current scientific understanding,[10] summarized here:

1. Safety first: anticipate potential danger to people and horses.

2. The horse: ensure his well-being by satisfying his needs and identifying potential causes of pain.

3. Your mood and state of mind: Don't let yourself be controlled by your emotions; keep in mind the mental and sensory capacities of horses, and don't jump to conclusions about their behavior.

4. Situation management: Prepare for situations you know are coming; pay attention to the horse's emotional state in the moment and identify it.

5. When the horse is afraid: Use habituation, desensitization, and calming techniques correctly.

6. Correct answers: use operant conditioning wisely, and know how to motivate the horse to try again if he engages in behavior you don't want.

7. Lightness: Use classical conditioning correctly, with precise, consistent cues.

8. Little by little: Teach behaviors reasonably—break complex behaviors down into the simplest possible steps for the horse.

9. Clarity: Make good use of signals and cues.

10. Autonomy: Allow the horse to move freely once a behavior has been learned—don't require what you don't need.

Dissecting the training of the horse, whether under saddle or as preparation for veterinary care, isn't easy to do in scientific terms, because it

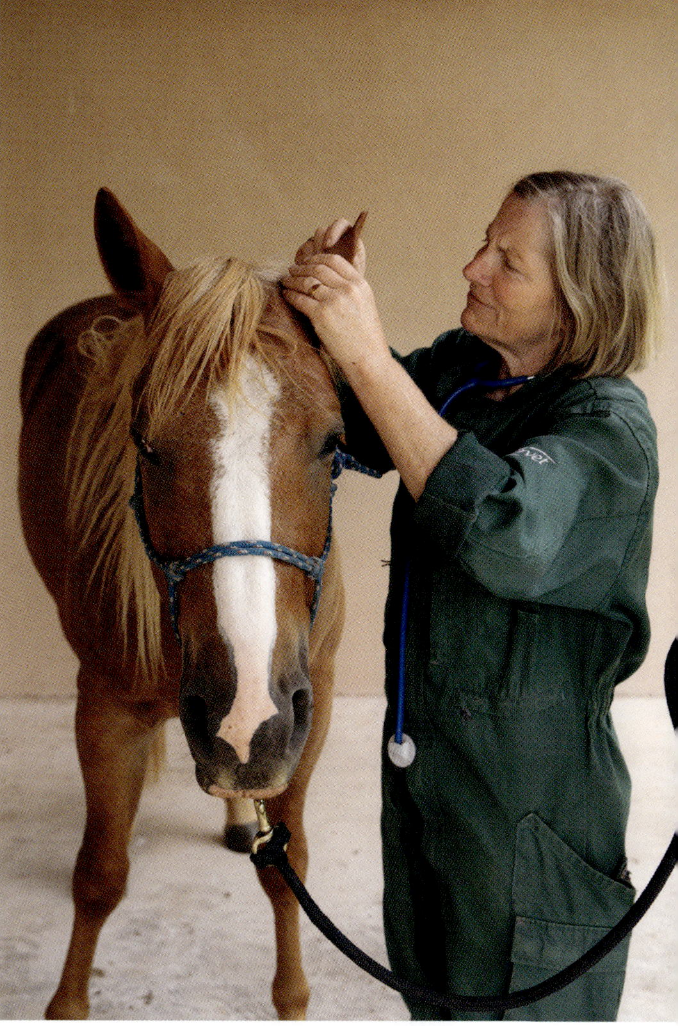

Point 10, autonomy: the horse is staying still during this examination of his ear, so there's no need to try to control his behavior further; the lead is hanging down, slack, and there's no extra tension being put on his head.

means using words and phrases that sound clinical. Some people find it an off-putting way to discuss our relationship with horses—they want to refer to feelings, to emotions. But in my opinion, a scientific approach and an emotionally sensitive approach aren't actually in opposition to each other; people who think of them as opposing perspectives often just don't fully understand whichever framing doesn't come naturally to them. Trying to apply learning theory without taking into account the individual equine we have in front of us, or our own emotions, doesn't work very well.

But, by the same token, relying solely on subjective feelings in the moment makes it difficult to share knowledge with other people or set standards for training, treatment, and care. Theories of learning framed with scientific terminology allow us humans to discuss what we're doing to improve our relationships with horses, ponies, and donkeys using a consistent and clearly defined vocabulary.

It's not that you need to use this vocabulary in order to be able to treat animals fairly; but it makes it easier to explain *how* to treat animals fairly— the principles of action involved, "what to do." This is the part I want to address when I bring up scientific theories and terminology.

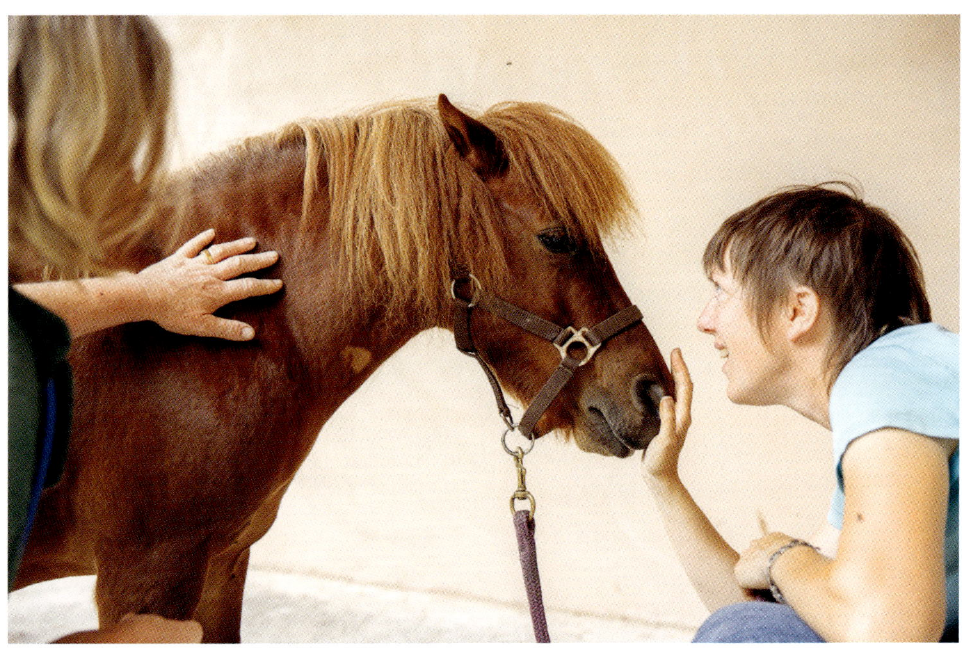

Even if horses can recognize the emotions on our human faces, that doesn't exempt us from putting in the effort to understand how learning theory applies to them. Emotion and science both matter.

Chapter 1

PREPARING IN ADVANCE

Taking care of an animal means, above all, taking steps to prevent problems and to respond to problems that do occur with a clear understanding of their causes.

Identifying Problems

Any change in behavior from whatever is normal for your horse, pony, or donkey is worth your attention. This can be anything from a sudden disinterest in you when he usually comes to greet you whenever you show up to uncharacteristic aggressiveness, or even a shift in his daily routine compared to the horses, ponies, or donkeys around him. If you find him sleeping at a time when he's usually active, and none of his friends and herdmates are resting, it's safest to check on him and make sure everything's okay. Refusing to eat is also a warning sign. Knowing what your animal looks, sounds, and acts like when everything is normal for him is a big help in spotting when there might be a problem—and most health issues only get more serious over time, so the earlier you can address them, the better. Spending time observing your horse, pony, or donkey, and taking notes or even photos on a regular basis gives you a "patient history" you can refer to if you need to. (One of my other books goes into more detail about the behaviors and activities you should monitor to track the well-being of your horse.[11])

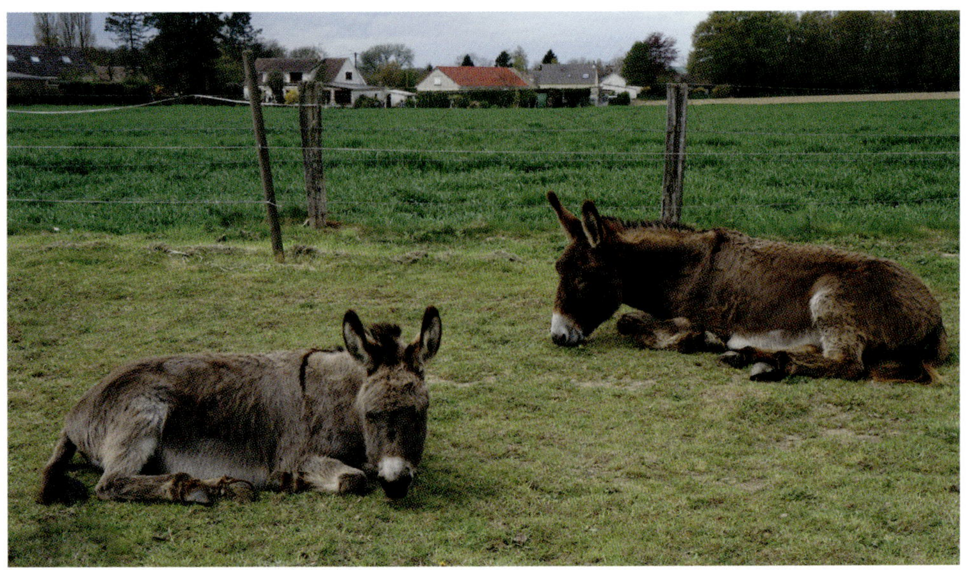

Lying down is normal for horses, ponies, and donkeys when they're sleeping, but an individual lying down for an unusually long time, or lying down when none of his herdmates are lying down, is a potential cause for concern.

Recognizing Pain in Horses or in Ponies

Pain, whether human or equine, is difficult to identify and difficult to objectively measure on a scale of severity. Humans and horses both have individual pain thresholds that affect how they react to pain. For example, during an episode of colic of exactly the same severity, a Thoroughbred will probably appear very agitated, rolling around or throwing himself to the ground, while a draft horse or a donkey will seem vaguely uncomfortable and decide to lie down quietly. So it's essential to get to know your individual horse, pony, or donkey well enough to tell what qualifies as a major pain response for him.

Aggression or agitation can signal the presence of pain, but so can prostration (lying down) with little or no reaction to outside stimuli. There are certain recognizable postures that some equines will adopt in order to relieve pain in one or more limbs, such as during an attack of laminitis in horses or ponies (though not typically in donkeys).

Various research has been done to try to create objective methods for assessing pain in horses, with the aim of making it easier to identify and relieve. Karina Gleerup and Casper Lindegaard[12] published a survey of multiple studies and proposed a scale to measure pain in horses based on behavioral characteristics (see the table on page 14).

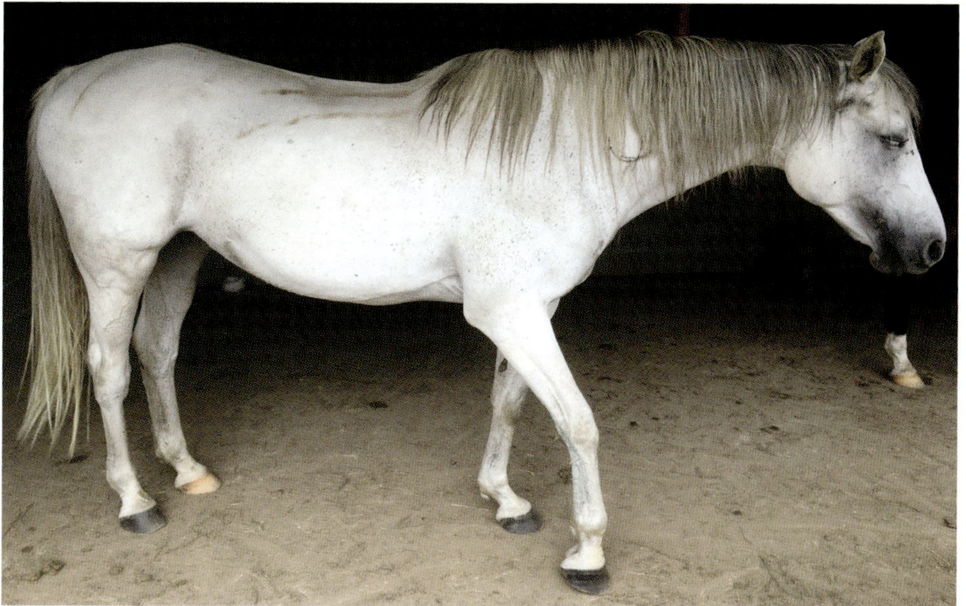

Unusual posture is often a sign of pain. Here, this mare is flexing her front leg in an atypical way while otherwise standing at rest, which is probably due to pain in her flexor tendons.

They chose not to include physiological metrics like heart rate or breathing rate, because those things depend to some degree on other factors in the horse's condition, and can't always be correlated with pain specifically. Evaluation using these metrics takes about two minutes. You may need to reassess your horse's pain multiple times during the day, or even hourly, depending on his condition. This system also includes a pain scale based on facial expression, which is described in more detail on the next few pages.

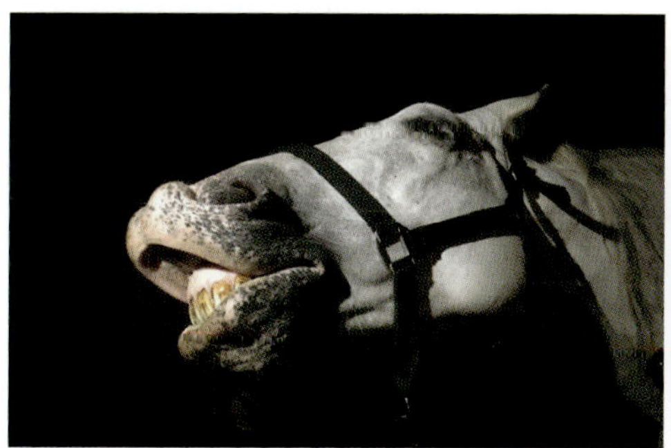

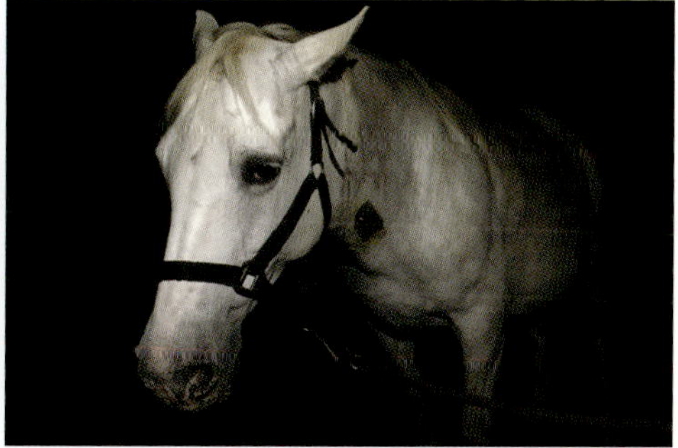

The *flehmen response* is often a reaction to an interesting smell, but it may also be performed repeatedly when a horse is in pain (left). Even without that response as a clue, observe the facial expression of this mare (right), who was presenting with multiple symptoms of colic.

	What You See with Horses and Ponies				
Category	0	1	2	3	4
Facial Expression Indicating Pain	Absent		Present	Intense	
Unusual Behaviors Indicating Pain*	None		Occasional		Continuous
Activity Level	Exploratory, interested in his surroundings or resting normally	Not moving		Agitated	Prostrated
Orientation in Stall**	Near the door, observing his surroundings	Standing in the middle of the stall, facing the door	Standing in the middle of the stall, facing a wall	Standing in the middle of the stall, facing away from the door; on the floor of the stall	
Posture and Distribution of Weight	Normal posture, weight distributed squarely on all four legs	Lifting a foot intermittently, or shifting weight occasionally (from left feet to right feet, or from front feet to back feet)	Tense (with contracted muscles, a visible furrow between the abdominal muscles, the stomach drawn in)	Keeping one foot consistently off the ground, trying to avoid any weight on it	Trying to avoid supporting his own weight as much as possible, or otherwise clearly abnormal distribution of weight
Head Position	Lowered normally to forage for hay or grass, raised if not eating	Held level with the back	Lowered even when he is not foraging		
Attention to Painful Area	No particular attention paid to potentially painful area		Brief attention to a potentially painful area (looking at his own flank sometimes, for example)		Biting or repeatedly touching a potentially painful area with the nose, looking at it constantly
Reaction to Observer	Looking at observer, coming to greet observer	Looking at observer without moving	Not looking at observer, or moving away to avoid contact	Not moving, not reacting at all	
Response to Food	Taking food without hesitation	Looking at the food, if not eating it right away		Not reacting to the presence of food	

Table 1: Equine pain scale, proposed by Karina Gleerup and Casper Lindegaard, explained by Hélène Roche.

* Unusual behaviors indicating pain include easily visible actions like excessive head movement (up and down or side to side), the flehmen response, kicking with the hindquarters (toward the abdomen or otherwise), pawing with the front feet, rolling, tail swishing, repetitive mouth movements (yawning, grinding the teeth), stretching, and so on. Please note that none of these behaviors, taken individually, are necessarily signs of pain; they'll also appear in other contexts.

** This row of observations is meant for horses in their stalls, but you can still assess horses in the paddock or the field by comparing their behavior to what's normal for them.

The work of Emanuella Dalla Costa and her colleagues[13] focuses on the facial expressions* of horses. They established a pain scale based on expression, using horses that had undergone castration surgery. There are six points in their assessment system:

- Orientation of the ears backward, and lack of movement in them;
- Lowering of the eyelid (closing the eyes);
- Degree of contraction in the muscle above the eye (the "eyebrow");
- Degree of contraction in the chewing muscles (the cheeks);
- Degree of tightness in the mouth and shape of the chin;
- Degree of contraction in the nostril and the flatness of its outline.

Each of these items is given a rating from 0 (absent or not at all) to 2 (completely), with 1 indicating an in-between state. It's possible for a horse's total score to be above zero even in the absence of pain, but it's a helpful indicator of a potential problem.

This facial expression assessment scale was tested on horses who had been castrated, horses with acute laminitis[14] (a vascular and necrotic disease** of the horse's feet that is very painful), and horses with dental

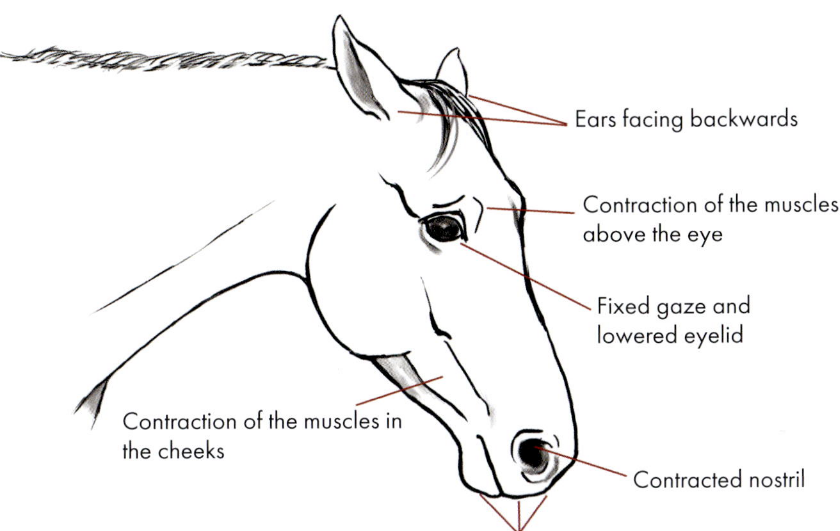

Expression of pain on the face of a horse, based on the work of Gleerup et al. (2015)

* I deliberately use the words "face" and "facial expression" here, which may seem like I'm anthropomorphizing. However, we discuss horses using words like "mouth," "nose," and "eyes," so why not call the sum of those things the "face"? Sometimes in scientific literature discussing horses, we refer to the horse's "head" rather than his "face." However, I think using "head" makes some people focus too much on the ears and the orientation of the head, and they don't pay enough attention to the details of the eyes, nostrils, and mouth. The word "face" encourages us to look at more than just the ears and head, and there's no real reason to avoid using it.

** "Necrotic" means a process of alteration that leads to the destruction of a cell or of organic tissue.

problems.[15] It hasn't been independently validated as an assessment for other painful conditions. In another study of the faces of horses feeling discomfort, this time induced using a cream with a strong warming effect and compression of the foreleg with a cuff as if to take the horses' blood pressure, the horses' eyelids were not lowered; on the contrary, they seemed to open their eyes wider cuff), horses were more interested in interacting with humans,[18] even though pain usually causes avoidance or aggression.[19] But there may be other factors involved—the horses in that study were with humans who were familiar to them and humans they strongly associated with food rewards, which may have encouraged them to seek contact instead of avoiding it. If that's what made the difference here,

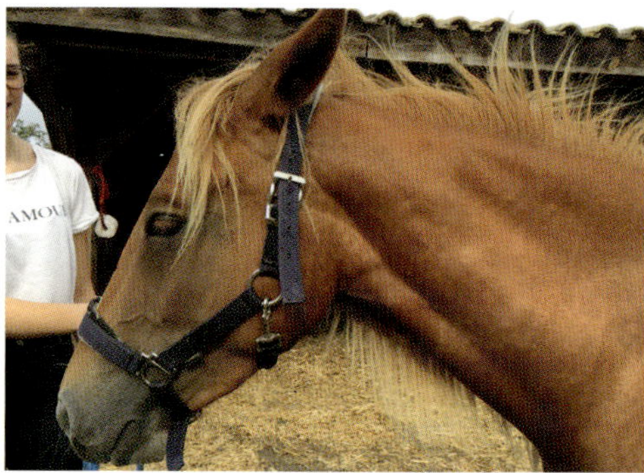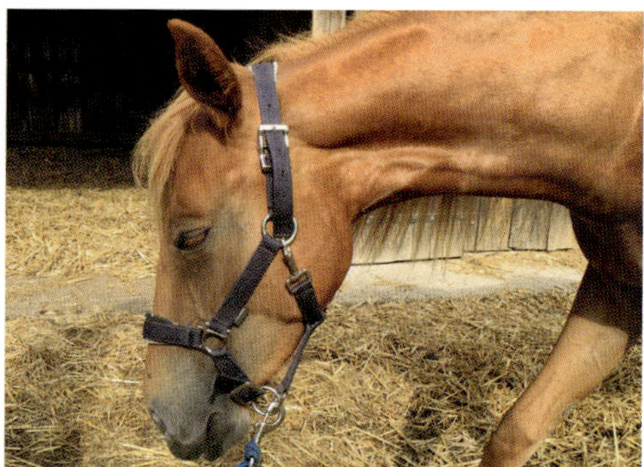

This pony was experiencing colic; her face expressed pain (left). Notice the change in her expression once she's sedated, especially the relaxation of her lips (right).

than usual, and gave the researchers the impression of a fixed, "intense" gaze[16] (the study's authors use "intense," a subjective term, to describe a reduction in the number of eyeblinks, which seemed to express worry, and eyes that were wide open but without the whites exposed[17]).

Some studies also give contradictory results at first glance when describing the reaction of horses in pain to humans. In some situations (for example, the experiment with the warming cream and blood pressure then that's good news for horses and their owners. The type of pain or discomfort the horse is experiencing may also affect his behavior toward humans, however, so in general, do not assume you can predict the reaction a horse, pony, or donkey will have toward you if he's in pain—he may look for contact, he may avoid it, or he may be aggressive. He also may not react the same way toward you as to someone else, like an unfamiliar vet.

With either of these systems for evaluating pain in horses, remember

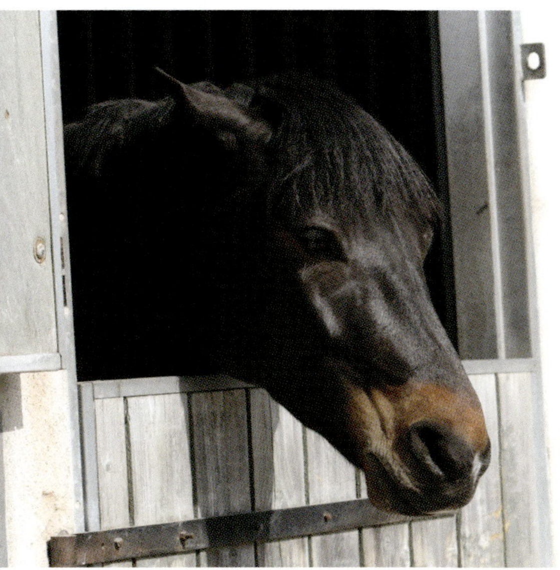

Aggression—here, the pinning of the ears as a threat to bite—can appear when an equine is in pain. Notice the narrow shape of the nostrils here, in comparison to the nostrils of the colicking pony on the facing page.

on its own, doesn't mean that pain is present. For example, a closed or half-closed eye is normal in a sleepy horse, and paying attention to one part of his body is perfectly normal for a horse who's got an itch.

If you use these assessments, keep their limitations in mind. At the very least, they're a good way to start training yourself to notice small changes in the posture or expression of a horse.

Recognizing Pain in Donkeys

Signs of illness and pain are usually more subtle in donkeys than they are in horses or ponies. Donkeys also tend to move less when they're worried or in pain, which makes it even more difficult to detect potential problems. However, recent research has identified indicators specific to donkeys. The overall assessment presented in the table on the next two pages should take less than five minutes.

that a horse who isn't in pain will not necessarily score a zero; a few assessments may come out at a 1. By the same token, a horse who *is* experiencing pain won't usually have a maximum score in every single category. Any one point on either scale,

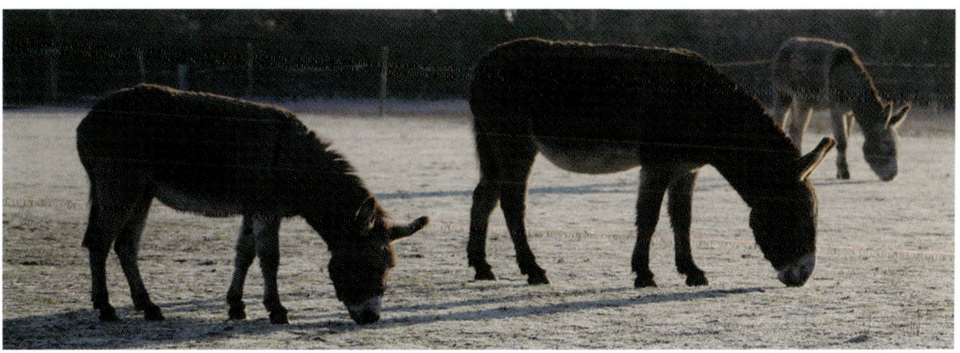

You have to observe the interactions of a donkey with the rest of his group in order to monitor his state of health accurately.

Category	What You See with Donkeys			
	0	1	2	3
General Appearance	Alert, willing to interact with companion or group	Slightly downcast/agitated, decreased interactions with companion or group	Downcast and/or aggressive and/or no interaction with companion or group	Severely downcast, no interest in interaction at all
Sounds Indicating Pain	No sounds	Occasional moaning or grinding of the teeth (1–2 times in 5 min)	Frequent moaning or grinding of the teeth (3–4 times in 5 minutes)	Excessive groaning or grinding of the teeth (>4 times in 5 min)
Change in Group Behavior	Part of the group			Companion or group has left or is moving away
Posture	Standing quietly, and/or with flexed hindquarters	Abdomen lifted slightly, and/or a slight change in weight distribution	Abdomen raised, and/or hunched back, and/or splayed legs, and/or muscle tremors	Sitting on hind legs and/or very pronounced muscle tremors
Distribution of Weight	Standing square with normal distribution of weight across all four legs			Uneven weight distribution
Head Position	Held so the bases of the ears are above withers, unless eating or drinking (from something on the ground)		Held so the bases of the ears are at the level of the withers	Held so the bases of the ears are lower than the line of the back
Rolling and Sleeping	Not lying down, or not staying down very long	Lying down or trying to lie down less than half the time	Lying down more than half the time	Lying down, in an abnormal position: on one side with legs outstretched, or on the back, or rolling repeatedly
Ear Position (More than 75% of the Time	Normal			Unusual (backwards, on their sides, flat)
Frequency of Tail Shaking (Other than to Remove Insects)	Not moving, tail in normal position	Occasional swishing of the tail (1–2 sessions in 5 min)	Frequent swishing of the tail (3–4 sessions in 5 min)	Excessive swishing of the tail (>4 sessions in 5 min), and/or lifting the tail or keeping the tail held between the buttocks
Interaction with Own Abdomen	No foot strikes toward or attention paid to own abdomen	Looking at own abdomen	Lifting a hind foot to strike own abdomen once or twice	Excessive striking of the abdomen (>2 times in 5 min)
Pawing the Ground	No pawing	Holding a forefoot forward as if about to paw	Occasional pawing (1–2 times in 5 min)	Frequent pawing (>2 times in 5 min)

Category	What You See with Donkeys			
	0	**1**	**2**	**3**
Reaction to Observer	Looking at and/or coming toward observer		Looking at observer without moving	Not moving, not reacting to observer at all
Response to Food	Taking food without hesitation		Eating less food, eating more slowly	No interest in food
Reaction to Palpation of Potentially Painful Area	No reaction		Moderate reaction	Strong reaction
Movement (Using Food to Motivate)	No reluctance to move, moving at normal pace	Slightly abnormal movement, and/or stiff gait	Reluctant to move when asked, and/or very awkward gait	Unwilling to move at all, lying down and not getting up

Table 2: The EQUUS-DONKEY COMPASS, adapted according to the recommendations of the authors.[20]

Donkeys often react to worry or pain with motionlessness, so using food to encourage them to move around is a good idea.[21] If the donkey isn't interested in food, asking his companion animal or group to move away from him in order to encourage him to follow them so you can evaluate his movement that way may also work. Donkeys can sometimes appear to be eating when they are actually only touching the food without consuming it, so you should use a "grip test," holding the food in your hand to see whether he's really pulling it into his mouth, to check.[22] The

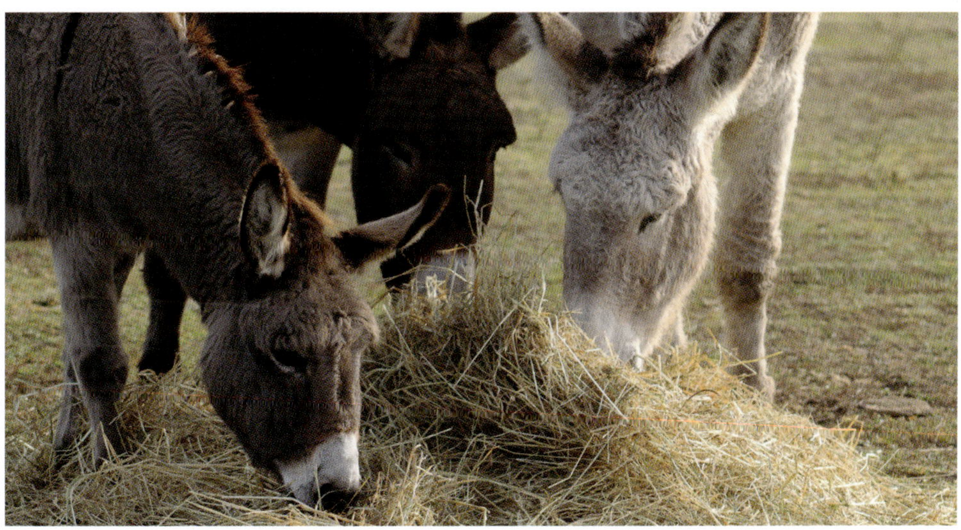

Donkeys sometimes give the illusion of eating when they are sick. You have to check their appetites by giving them food by hand to see whether they are actually eating it.

overall assessment of a donkey's pain in Table 2 can be supplemented with a donkey-specific pain rating scale for facial expressions. Here's a combination of two facial expression rating scales that have been tested in donkeys—it should take about two minutes to complete. Each of the items is given a rating from 0 (absent or not at all) to 2 (completely), with 1 indicating an in-between state.

- Abnormal positioning of the ears (see details below);
- Lack of reaction to noise (from 0, indicating a clear reaction with both ears, or with the ear closest to the source of the noise, to 2, no reaction to noise at all, with 1 indicating a reduced or delayed reaction);
- Lowering of the eyelid (closing the eye), or, conversely, opening the eye so far the sclera is visible;
- Contraction of the facial muscles (fasciculations*);
- "Inward" gaze (from 0, gaze focused on the environment, to 2, no attention to the environment);
- Tightening of the mouth and lips;
- Flehmen responses, or yawning and chewing;
- Contracted nostrils with visible wrinkles, and potentially audible breathing;
- Grinding of the teeth, moaning, or both.

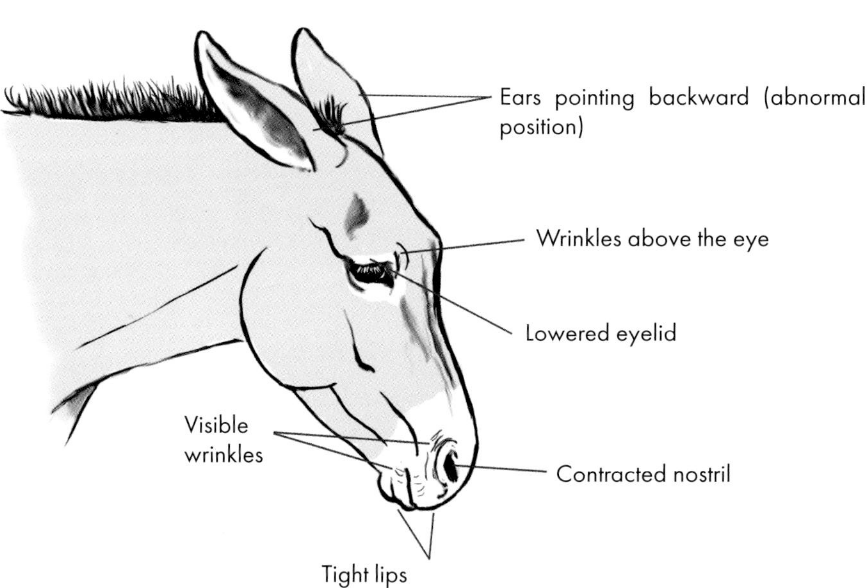

Indications of pain in the facial expression of a donkey, based on the work of Burden, F. & Thiemann, A. (2015), and Orth et al. (2020).

* Fasciculation: the brief involuntary contraction of a group of muscle fibers, visible when observing the skin.

The paper by Emma Orth[24] and her colleagues is the most detailed in describing abnormal positions for donkeys' ears. Ear positions that may be a sign of pain or discomfort include: both ears facing rearward, both ears to the side and facing downward, one ear forward and one ear down, one ear to the side and the other facing rearward, and one ear to the side and the other facing downward (see diagrams below).

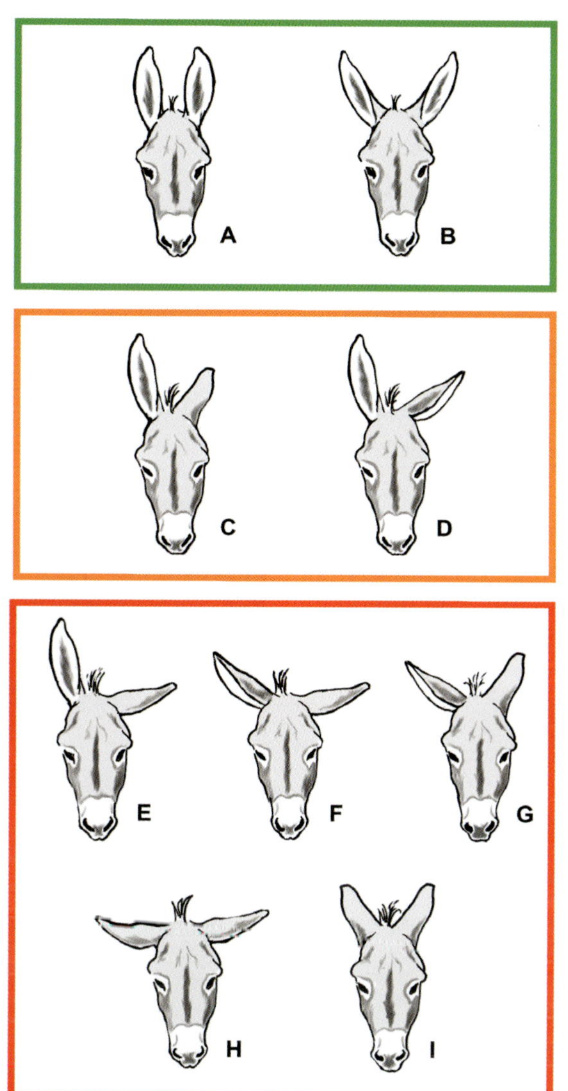

Descriptions of ear positions linked to pain in donkeys, according to Orth et al. (2020).
Rarely a sign of pain: both ears positioned facing forward (A), or raised and facing slightly sideways (B).
Sometimes a sign of pain: one ear facing forward and the other facing backward (C), or one ear facing forward and the other facing sideways (D).
Often a sign of pain: one ear facing forward and one ear lowered and facing downward (E), one ear to the side and one lowered and facing downward (F), one ear to the side and one facing backward (G), both ears lowered and facing downward (H), and both ears facing backward (I).

With acute orthopedic pain (laminitis, abscess) or following surgical castration, table 2 (pages 18–19) which assesses overall condition and behavior, is a better choice for evaluation than the facial pain scale, because signs are more likely to show in the body and posture. With pain occurring on or near the head (dental problems, uveitis, corneal ulcers, eye injuries), facial expressions will be more reliable.[25] For a donkey experiencing colic, both assessments will show a level of acute, visceral pain.

As for horses, the authors note that, with donkeys, pain assessment scales based on behavior or facial expressions are meaningful in and of themselves, even if you haven't taken any physiological data[26] (rectal temperature, heart rate, respiratory rate, sweating, or observations of digestive sounds—except for the last, which is an important diagnostic in cases of colic).

The assessment of chronic pain in equines hasn't been formally studied yet.

Identifying Fear in Horses, Ponies, Donkeys, or Mules

An animal won't cooperate, and may even resist treatment, if he doesn't understand what's expected of him or he's afraid. Confusion in and of itself can make animals frustrated or afraid—and, faced with this situation, we tend to react by adding more physical restraints and handling the animal more roughly, which only serves to make him more confused and more afraid. So identifying what fear looks like in equines is crucial; that way, you can tell when the individual animal you're working with is starting to become afraid, and you can adjust your approach until his fear has eased or gone away. As with pain, any individual expression or behavior that might be a sign of fear isn't necessarily conclusive in and of itself—it's the sum of these signs, how much the animal is repeating them, and how emphatic they are that will tell you whether he's afraid and how afraid he is.

With a horse who's afraid, you'll notice various signs in his body:

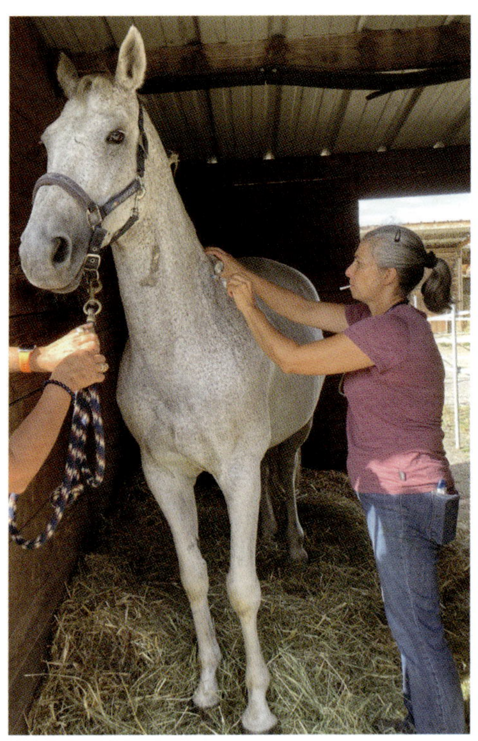

The raising of the neck reflects concern in the horse.

 — PREPARING YOUR HORSE OR DONKEY FOR VETERINARY CARE

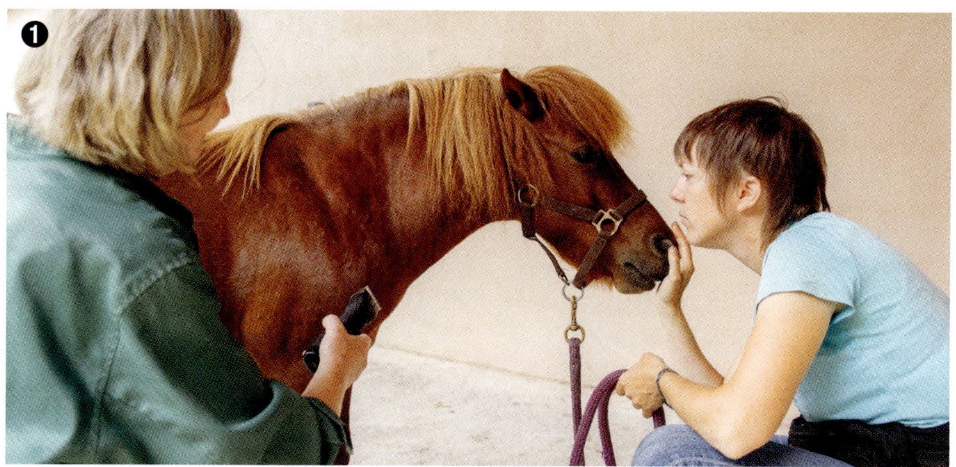

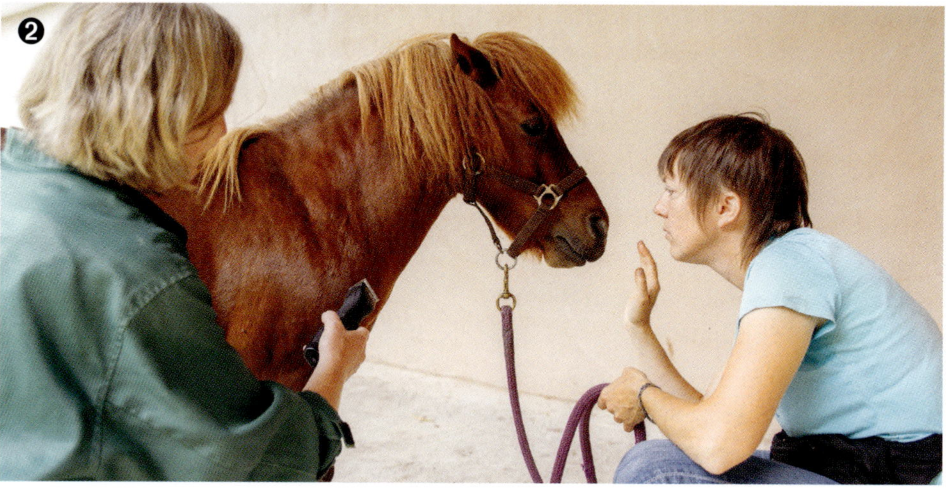

The pony, who at first is willing to lean on my hand ❶, breaks contact and raises his neck, widening his eyes without blinking ❷. We need to slow down here, since he's telling us he's not ready to accept the clippers held by the vet.

- An overall tension, with raising of his neck and tail if he's preparing to move away. If he's very frightened, on the other hand, his tail may be pressed between his buttocks instead of raised or extended, and in cases of extreme fear, he will bend his hocks.

- Avoidant movements of his head or body (turning away, backing up, or moving forward, trying to avoid handling, or even rearing if other movements are impossible).

- An increased level of movement, or, conversely, little to no movement, as if he's frozen in place.

- A tense mouth with tight lips.

- Wide eyes, with little to no blinking; if he's very frightened, the whites of his eyes may be showing.

- Ears pointed in the direction of his attention—whether that's very mobile because he's looking for his friends, or pointed fixedly forward, or pinned back toward the rear.

He may also make sounds:

- Neighing, with his mouth open, neck straight, and tail raised, if he's worried about being separated from his buddies and trying to figure out where they are.
- Snorting or blowing if he has noticed an object or noise that worries him—if he wants to move away from it but can't, he'll actively make these sounds instead.

There are also visible physiological signs of fear in horses:

- Repeated defecation, with less and less mass each time, and more and more liquid matter.
- Accelerated heart rate and breathing rate—to the point where it may be comparable to a horse at a gallop, even though this horse is standing still.
- Sudden sweating in the absence of physical exertion or fever, enough so that sweat may be dripping from him.

In donkeys, the most common response to fear is immobility. If this gets ignored and the handler keeps trying to make the donkey do something, the donkey may then turn to defensive behaviors: kicking or biting, for example. Donkeys are particularly quick to kick forward with their hindquarters, and if they can't escape the situation, they may also try to pin their handler against a solid object—so identifying fear in donkeys before it reaches this point helps reduce risk for the humans around them. Changes in facial expression are worth paying attention to, although they'll vary depending on the donkey:

- Nostrils tensed or closed.
- Tense nose and mouth, and particularly the chin and lips, which will create lots of visible folds and small wrinkles around these areas.
- A change in the cast of the eye, and a tense upper eyelid; sometimes donkeys also open their eyes wide enough to show more of the sclera (more of the white, especially at the upper part of the eye, than usual).[27]

Mules behave like a cross between donkeys and horses, appropriately enough. Their signs of fear may seem subtle, if you're used to working with horses, and they are usually quicker to switch to flight or defense than donkeys, which has earned them a reputation for being explosive and violent.

Identifying Relaxation and Calm in Horses and Ponies

It's just as important to be able to spot signs of relaxation as signs of fear—being able to tell that the animal you're working with is relaxed lets you continue examining him or providing care without worry. A relaxed horse shows signs such as:

- Holding his neck at a level that matches the line of his back, horizontal instead of raised (or holding his head below the height of the tourniquet, if he's sedated).

- Holding his ears facing downward, or allowing them to move apart.
- If he's standing still, allowing his tail to lie against his buttocks, but not pressing it between them; if he's walking, holding it slightly raised.
- Having his eyes open, or half-closed at most, and blinking regularly.
- Keeping his mouth relaxed, with a lower lip that sags or even hangs slightly open.
- Flexing a hind leg, or allowing it to rest in a slightly bent position with the toe of his hoof against the ground.
- Standing still calmly.
- For a male horse, whether he's a gelding or not, allowing his penis to protrude.

Identifying Impatience in Horses, Ponies, and Donkeys

What is often taken for impatience in an equine ("He's fed up!") is actually more likely to be a sign of either fatigue or pain. Responding by increasing the degree of restraint he's under, or rushing to try to finish up with him more quickly, is not usually a good idea. Look for signs such as:

- The animal starting to move around, if he was willingly standing still, or moving more than he was before;
- Swishing of the tail;
- Pawing with a foreleg;
- Accelerated breathing;

- Sweating;
- Starting to make noise;
- Increasingly tense or raised posture.[29]

If you spot these, it's time to give the animal a break, and release him from any physical restraints. If you don't, you're probably going to see increasingly intense and dangerous behaviors (striking, lateral hind kick, rearing, fleeing, jumping, and so on).

Preparing for a Vet Check at the Barn

Horses and donkeys are usually lucky, and get to stay in a familiar environment for a vet check—unlike our dogs and cats, who typically have to go to the vet's office. Even for advanced examinations like medical imaging (x-rays, ultrasounds, endoscopies), technology has progressed to the point where most equine veterinarians are able to carry mobile equipment. But even though the horse is often in a familiar place, we shouldn't underestimate his reactions to the parts of the process that are new to him: to being examined by a less familiar or even unknown person, and to unusual movements and gestures. Think again about the location where your horse gets examined by the vet. Is it truly well-known to him? If you remove your horse from his paddock for an examination, even if the examination is happening right next to that paddock, he's not necessarily going to feel calm—not if he usually walks past the paddock on his way in or out, instead of stopping there to be poked and prodded.

If you want to give the horse as little reason to be agitated as possible, then he has to have been trained to stand still and stay calm in the place where he'll be examined—for example, through grooming sessions in the same location. Also, consider the context of his vet check. If your horse is never alone in his paddock, but the vet check means his friends have been herded away, or they're all still in the paddock but he's been taken to the stable for the vet check, then he might be very worried before the examination has even started. If the vet agrees to it and there are no safety concerns, consider letting him stay in his paddock. It's also better to hold the horse than to tie him, unless he needs to go into a stock. Choose a place he knows, where he feels safe, with as little disturbance as possible around him (minimal noise, minimal passersby). If the horse is calm from the beginning, you'll be starting the examination off on the right note. For donkeys, specialists in the field recommend that his favorite buddy or usual companion animal be there during a vet check, to encourage him to stay responsive[30] instead of freezing with worry, which would make an examination or diagnosis a lot more difficult for the vet.

Once an examination has started, the vet is going to be using

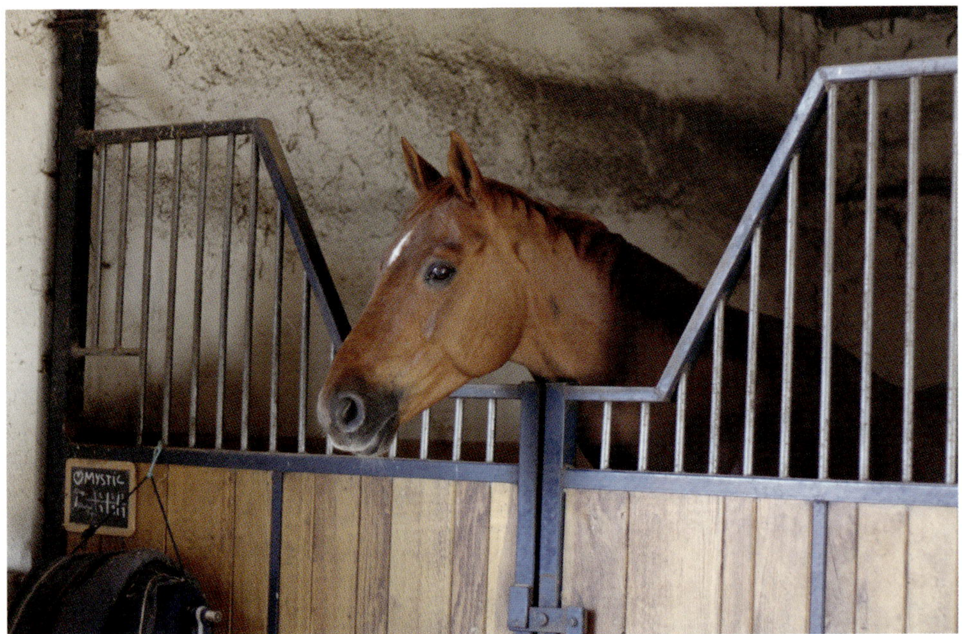

If all his friends are in the paddock and he alone has been taken to the stable for a vet check, your horse might be worried right off the bat. Help him stay calm with a buddy standing nearby to reassure him.

 —— PREPARING YOUR HORSE OR DONKEY FOR VETERINARY CARE

instruments that create stimuli for all of an equine's senses: they make noise, sometimes just from impact even when we're just setting them down; they have unusual shapes (think of a stethoscope, which as far as an animal is concerned is connected to the vet with a pipe and is suddenly reaching for his body); they are often reflective; they feel unusual (cold, for metallic instruments; slick, for an ultrasound probe; vibrating, for clippers; or simply unfamiliar, like the touch of a hand in a rubber glove); they give off strange odors… The vet will also move around in ways that may surprise your horse, pony, or donkey. And having two humans nearby instead of just one may also make him worry. We'll be discussing how to train an equine to stay relaxed in the face of all of these different situations and sensations.

Preparing for a Vet Check at the Clinic

Sometimes it might be necessary to take your horse, pony, or donkey to the clinic, instead of having the vet come to you. An emergency scenario with severe colic potentially needing surgery is probably the first thing that leaps to mind, but there are less dramatic cases where you might still have to take an equine to the vet that don't involve hospitalization. Vet clinics sometimes have diagnostic equipment that can't be moved but is needed for supplemental examinations, or

there may be other procedures that need to take place on-site. So there's every chance that your horse, pony, or donkey might need to go to the clinic one day—an event involving transport, arrival in a new location, and potentially a great deal of handling by unfamiliar people (additional vets, veterinary assistants, and so on) in uncomfortable circumstances. In addition, your equine is going to be separated from his pasture-mates, and if he isn't used to it, that will worry him. He might have to enter an examination room, a relatively enclosed and sometimes small space, often with few or no windows. If he has to wait his turn, or if the exam requires it, he may also end up in an unfamiliar stall.

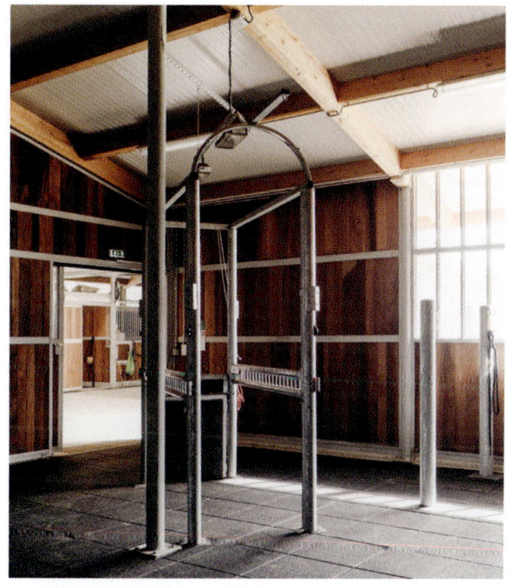

Both shadows cast on the ground and bright spots of light are visually disconcerting to horses. You have to let them lower their heads so they can inspect it before they have to step over it, or they'll want to stop, back away, or jump instead.

For purposes of hygiene, and to reduce the risk of disease transmission between equines while they're at the vet, this kind of stall usually has three solid walls, and the animal is only able to look out over the door—unless there's a grille instead of an open front, in which case it's more like having *four* solid walls, for him. It's common for the veterinary staff at the clinic to be responsible for caring for the animal, and for all examinations to be carried out without you around.

In this situation, it's easy to see there are lots of potential sources of stress for your animal. Each requires training to prepare for. You don't have to actually take your equine to a clinic to train him in advance, but

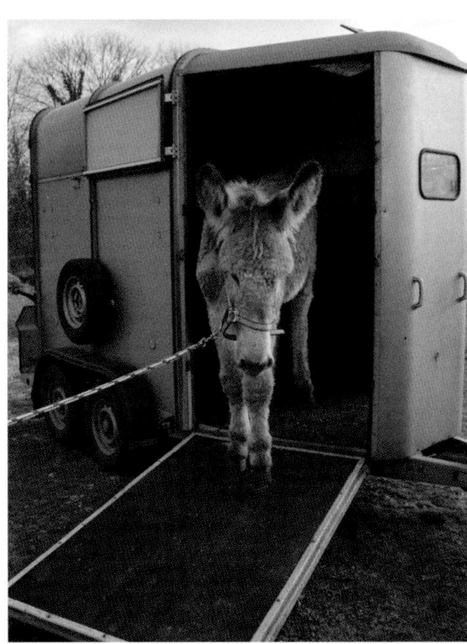

Training an equine to travel is important to avoid additional stress during an emergency situation.

loading him into a trailer and taking him to other kinds of unfamiliar places will make it a lot easier for him to adjust to new environments in general. Competitions, hacking out, and trail rides in a group are all great opportunities to work on this. As a bonus, these activities also involve separating your equine from his friends and pasture-mates, which will help him understand that being away from them doesn't pose a danger to him. It's up to you to focus on making sure transportation and being away from the barn are pleasant experiences, so he can develop positive associations with them. If you only ever trailer him to take him to places he doesn't like to do things he doesn't want to do, he'll only grow more reluctant to travel. And if the only times he's transported anywhere are medical emergencies where he's in pain, you're more likely to have trouble getting him into the truck or trailer, thanks to illness, injury, or discomfort, and you're *definitely* giving him negative associations with transportation.

To train your equine to enter a stall and stay there if he's not used to doing it, take advantage of the opportunities you get during other activities with him. The first time you take him into a stall, take him out again without leaving him there; then, take him in, reward him with a piece of carrot or something else he enjoys and let him eat it in the stall, and let him out again. If he's reluctant to go in at all, reward him for each step in

 — PREPARING YOUR HORSE OR DONKEY FOR VETERINARY CARE

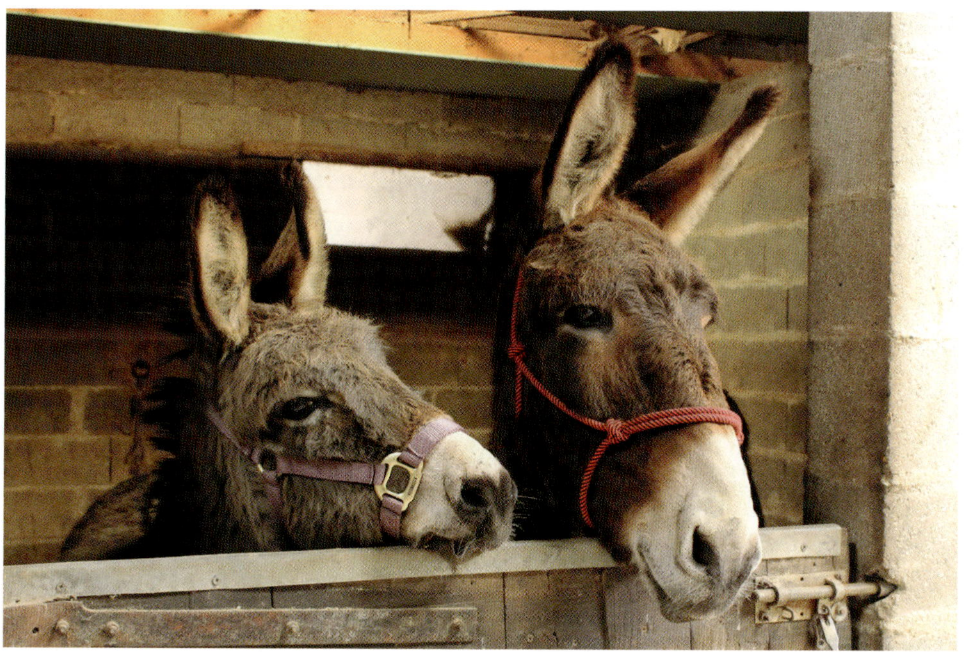

For a donkey or horse that hasn't been kept in a stall very much, the presence of a friend can help reassure him. This is especially recommended for donkeys.

the right direction. Once he can enter the stall and he is relaxed about it, let him wait for a few seconds inside, and then extend this time. As you continue, you can put a bucket with his food inside the stall, to give him a reason to want to be there.

You can also ask him to go in, and then close the stall, having shown him in advance that you put a few pieces of carrot or apple (depending on what he likes and what you have to hand) in various places around the stall, to encourage him to explore it as he eats. This way, you can train your horse, pony, or donkey to stay calm in a stall. And if a calm neighbor is in the next stall over, that will make this process even easier.

If you're usually the only person who handles your equine, take advantage of visits from your friends and family to let him get used to being approached by new people. Having someone unfamiliar take him for a walk in-hand or groom him a little is enough.

Working on this kind of training regularly is important. If you get your horse used to living in a stall and being separated from his friends, and then several months or years go by where he's living in a paddock with a group, if you don't keep training him, then when he's confronted with a stall by himself, he's going to get worried all over again. A quick reminder every couple of months is enough, as long as you stick with it.

We'll cover training for specific veterinary procedures in the next few chapters.

Preparing for a Hospitalization or Long-Term Immobilization

Preparing your horse to stay in a stall should be included in your training program in general, as discussed above.

"Hospitalization" doesn't necessarily mean your equine will be staying at a clinic. It's possible for animals, just as it is for humans, to be on "bed rest" at home. This is potentially the case for horses who don't need very much day-to-day care, but have to stay strictly immobilized in the stable—for example, for a suspected or proven fracture, or serious damage to a tendon. During this kind of hospitalization, the length of his confinement and the lack of stimulation are going to be unpleasant for your animal. It's a good idea to enrich his environment with safe physical and sensory opportunities.

Here are some possibilities that may be appropriate, if your vet agrees:

- Add hay nets to his stall (if he's allowed to eat when he wants to), though they should be removed at night if he has shoes in order to make sure he can't get a shoe caught in the net while no one is around. Even with unlimited hay on the floor of his stall, adding hay nets creates variation in the height and location he's feeding at;

- Attach a support where he can scratch himself (a brush or a door-mat with a scratchy texture, on the wall);

- Hide pieces of carrot or edible fruits and vegetables in his pile of hay (apple pieces, orange slices, artichoke leaves, pieces of banana peel or fruit, pineapple pieces, plum pieces, cherries, blackberries), or other edible forage like dandelion flowers and leaves, varying the treat and observing to see which ones he likes the best;

- Give him something to smell (soak a cotton ball with a few drops of an essential oil and put it in an open plastic bottle, out of reach of the horse's mouth, swapping smells regularly—but check in advance to make sure there's no contraindications with a treatment in progress for him, or for other animals in nearby stalls);

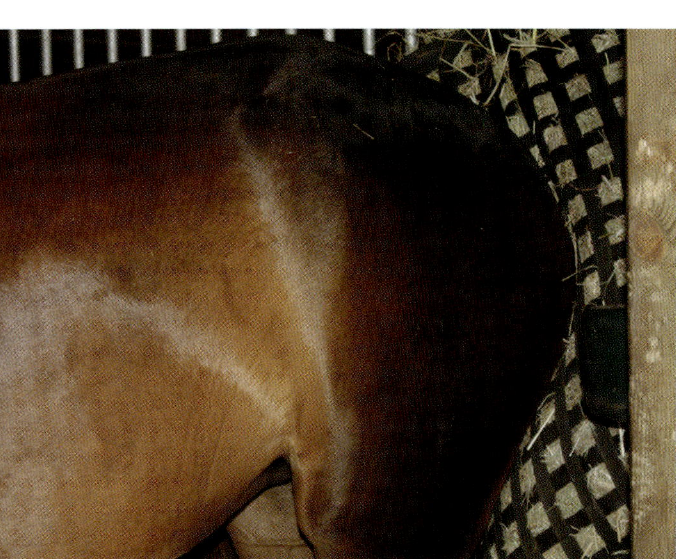

A hay net also slows down the eating process so it takes longer and fills up more of a bored equine's time—and it can serve as an improvised scratching post, too.

- Bring him new objects he can safely explore and play with (large dog toys are generally good candidates)—give him one for a few days, and then remove it and replace it with a new one, rotating items without switching back to the first one until at least ten days have passed so he stays interested in them);
- Take him for short outings in-hand, if his condition allows it;
- Give him some grooming and scratching sessions.

Environmental enrichment for confined equines reduces the frequency of stereotypies (repetitive behaviors without any apparent purpose, like cribbing or weaving), and it makes caring for them easier, in comparison to horses who are confined and only get to interact with anything new during examinations or feeding times.[31] Above and beyond making confinement easier, the benefits of enrichment for the relationship between humans and horses has been demonstrated with yearlings.[32]

Horses can also be cognitively stimulated. What I mean by "cognitive stimulation" is giving him something to think about or figure out—like teaching him exercises using positive reinforcement, in particular with the techniques of clicker training. There are some behaviors you can ask for even when the horse has to stand still, so they're readily compatible with stall rest or even immobilization, when the horse can only move his head, ears, nose, neck, and at most one foot. I'll cover the basics of clicker training in the next few chapters.

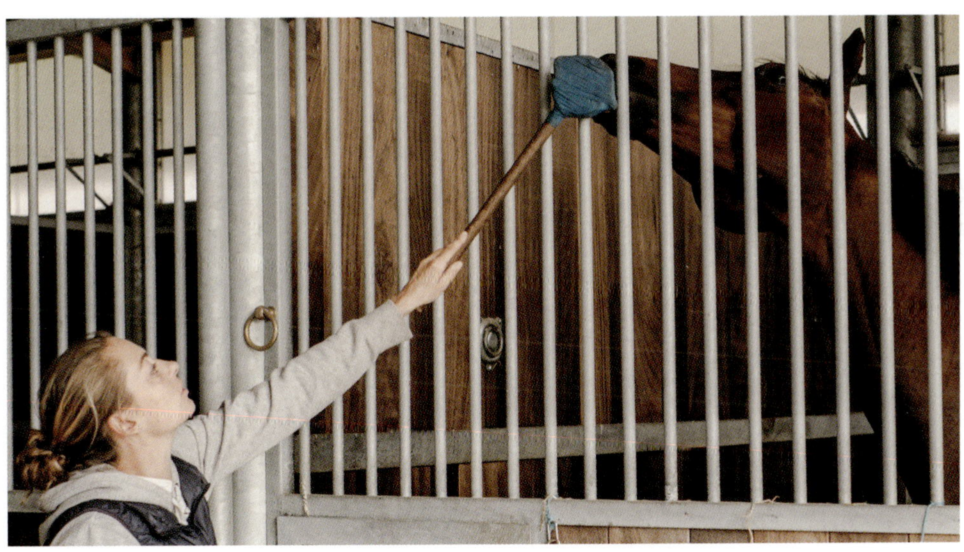

Learning to touch a target and follow it is great cognitive stimulation for a confined or immobilized horse. It also helps him maintain positive relationships with humans. The "Touch-Click" exercise is described on page 47.

This cognitive stimulation benefits the horse's well-being, and it also makes him more cooperative during sometimes-painful treatments—if, for example, he has uveitis[33] (a very painful eye condition). For donkeys, specialists in the field recommend that their favorite buddy or most consistent companion animal be present, to help the sick or injured donkey cope better with treatment. Separation leads some donkeys to stop eating or drinking, which puts their health even more seriously at risk than the original medical issue.[34]

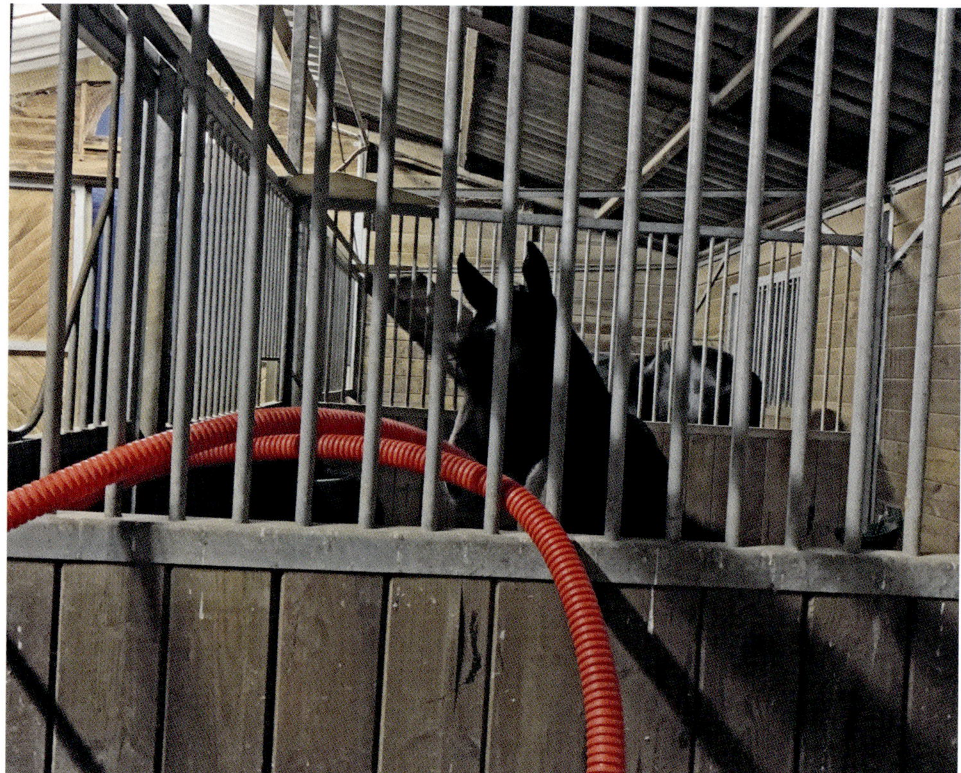

In the case of this foal, who was confined to a stall, this plastic conduit tubing enriched his environment considerably. He could bite the tubes, pull on them (which produced a noise as they bumped against the stall bars), rub against their textured surfaces, or even trample on them if he pulled them down far enough. They were safe for him: there was no risk that he could bite through the material and ingest a piece, he would not hurt his foot by stepping on them, and the relative rigidity of this kind of tubing meant they couldn't get wrapped around his neck (so there was no risk of strangulation).

Chapter 2

THE BASICS: TEACHING STILLNESS AND MANAGING REWARDS

Using methods of restraint that can cause pain, like twisting an ear with your hand or using a twitch,[35] is strongly discouraged. However, I'll still discuss both restraint by the ear and with a twitch, as these methods unfortunately can't always be discarded as options, even though the aim of this book is to reduce the need for them, and to eliminate it altogether wherever possible. In order to do this, I strongly encourage you to train your horse, pony, donkey, or mule to stand still on his own, in all kinds of situations. That will make it much easier for you to request other behaviors from him while he's receiving veterinary care,

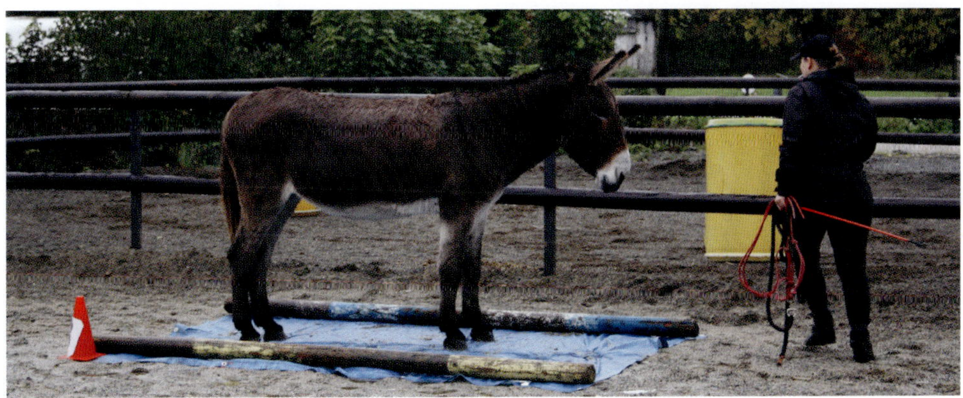

Thanks to his training, this donkey readily stands still during an exercise in competition. This skill will be very useful when he needs veterinary care.

and allow you to avoid unnecessary restraints, too. Staying still is a matter of both understanding the animal's perspective and simply being patient. Having an animal stand still for as long as you ask can be taught. Don't expect your horse to stay still for five minutes straight if you haven't prepared him for it, and lower your expectations further when he's worried or in pain. Likewise, don't expect your horse to accept food rewards calmly if you haven't taught him what I call "politeness"— he won't know any better.

In my opinion, in any case other than an emergency situation, you have to put some rules in place for your equine when it comes to food rewards. For an emergency, skip this step and go straight to the instructions for the technique you need; you can come back and teach "manners" another time.

To start off on the right foot with food rewards, I recommend you use clicker training, which is based on positive reinforcement. It involves indicating to your animal when he has done the right thing by giving him a signal (these exercises will describe the noise of the clicker as the signal, but you can substitute a word, or a click of your tongue) at the exact moment he shows the correct behavior, and then giving him a food reward. Patting can be reassuring and comforting, but is not nearly as motivating for this kind of training; scratching can work, but is less effective,[36] except for some individual animals who love it and for foals up to the age of about a year, since they're not used to accepting rewards given by hand. To familiarize yourself with this technique so you can teach the horse to manage his excitement and frustration over food, start with the exercises on the following pages.

- Help your animal get used to the sound of the clicker so it doesn't scare him, with the Click-Treat exercise;

- Teach him the good manners I've grouped under the term "politeness," with the Statue, Hand in the Bag, and Switching Sides exercises;

- Go further, with the Touch-Click exercise.

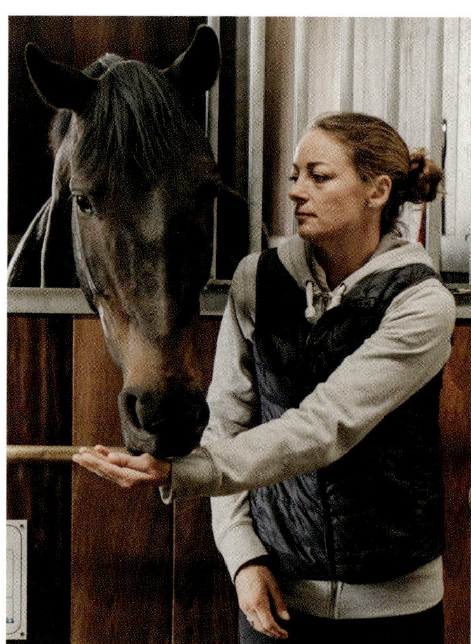

Managing excitement over the presence of food, and frustration over having it temporarily withheld, can be taught and trained.

Just Click

What's the Point?

Training an animal means putting yourself in the role of the teacher. Before teaching anything to your student, the horse, you should make sure you understand what you're going to do and how you're going to do it. This exercise has you practice clicking at the right moment without the horse around—not a moment before the behavior you want to reward, and not the moment after, but at the same time. This is what we call "temporal contiguity," in scientific terms. Practicing this will develop your focus and coordination with the clicker, without letting you confuse the horse with mistakes as you learn the technique.

What You're Practicing

- Clicking to signal a reward at the right time.

✦ What You Do

For this exercise, ask someone to be your partner, or even do it in a group. One person should have a ball, either one that bounces or one they can toss (either from one of their own hands to the other, or to another person in the group). Have them bounce or toss the ball, and try to click the clicker at the exact moment the ball hits the ground or lands in the hand of whoever is catching it. At first, keep the pace slow and steady so you can keep up; then, if you're comfortable with your timing, have the ball handler(s) go faster, and less predictably. You can also practice variations like clicking as someone walks in front of you—for example, every time their left heel touches the ground. They can also hop, jump, and shuffle, in between normal steps, to keep you guessing and test your clicking skills.

Common Mistakes

- Clicking multiple times instead of just once;
- Clicking before the ball hits the ground/a hand;
- Forgetting to click at all;
- Clicking at the wrong moment (when the right heel touches down, in our example, instead of the left heel).

Click-Treat

What's the Point?

Some of you have probably already been wondering whether the noise of a clicker (or any other signal you've chosen) might frighten your horse,

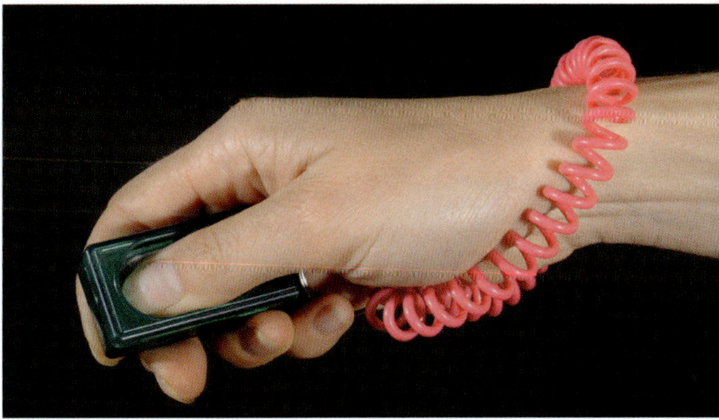

A clicker emits a sound your horse will learn to associate with a reward.

pony, or donkey—and you're right to wonder! The first thing you should do, once you're ready to work with your horse instead of on your own, is let the horse get used to the sound (scientifically, this is the phenomenon of *habituation**). If your horse is already used to the sound of you clicking your tongue, or whatever other signal you've picked, then this exercise is not as important; but it can still be helpful to teach both you and your horse to associate a click with a reward.

What You're Practicing

- Giving a reward consistently and correctly;
- Getting in the habit of giving a reward after clicking.

What You Want the Horse to Do

- Get used to the sound of the clicker.
- Form an association between the click and a food reward.

✦ What You Do

To stop the horse from going through your pockets, and to avoid having to push him away, choose a place for this where the horse is on one side of a barrier and you're on the other (on opposite sides of a gate in a paddock fence, a stall door, an arena wall, or the fence of a round pen). *Don't* use an electric fence for this—if your horse is already wary of it, he won't want to approach, even for a treat; and if he isn't, then he'll learn to be in short order if he touches it to reach for his treat at the wrong time. Plus, the sound of the clicker might remind a horse who's familiar with electric fences of the sound of the shocks they give.

1. Take the clicker in one hand, sliding it into your pocket to muffle the sound;

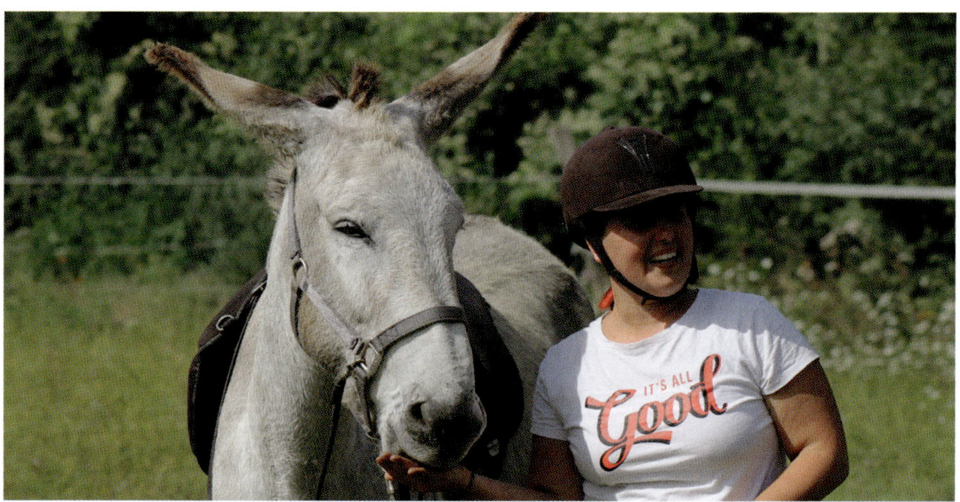

At first, you might forget to extend your arm to give your animal a treat. The point is to make it a very deliberate motion—to establish that we're giving the treat to the animal, rather than the animal coming to get the treat on his own initiative.

2. Click, and then use your free hand to give the horse a treat.

3. Repeat 1–3 times, and if the horse is no longer showing any signs of concern over the noise (blowing, backing up, moving away):

4. Take the clicker out of your pocket and hold it behind your back;

5. Click, and use your hand to give a treat with each click, at least three times.

6. Then hold the clicker at your side, with your arm hanging straight down, and click, rewarding after each click, repeating at least three more times.

Reach out to the horse to give him his reward—you're the one giving it to him, so he shouldn't be coming to you to take it. You can even take a step toward him to give it to him, and then return to place. This will cement the idea for both of you: you are going to give the reward, and the horse should stay where he is and wait for it to be given to him (not go looking for it!).

Common Mistakes

- Leaving your free hand in the treat bag all the time;
- Putting your free hand in the treat bag before clicking;
- Pointing the clicker at the horse when you click;
- Giving the horse the treat with the same hand that is holding the clicker.

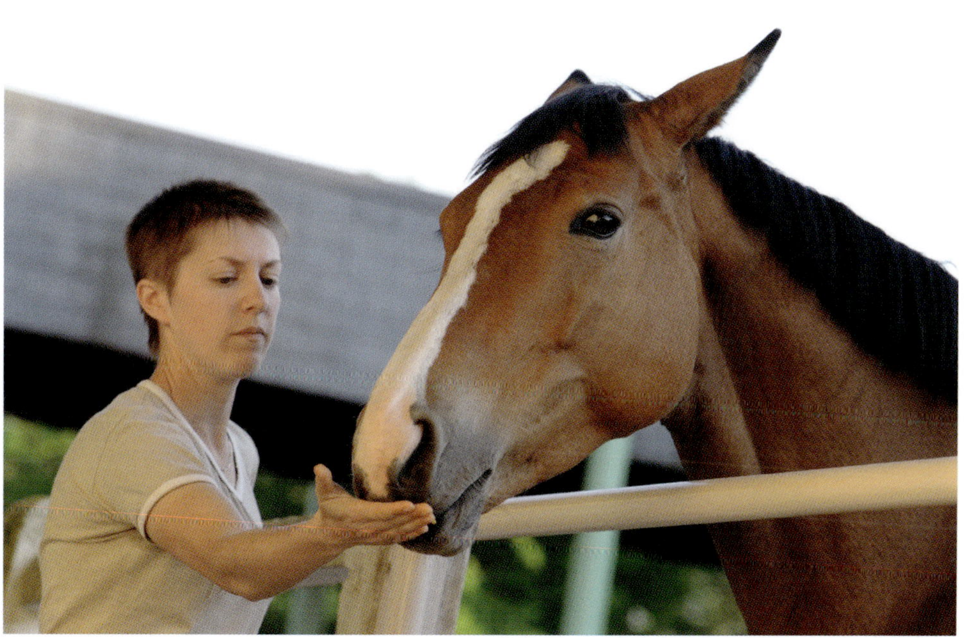

Remember to move toward the animal and extend your arm to give him the treat.

*See the glossary on page 171.

The Statue

What's the Point?

This exercise is about teaching the horse that when you're next to him, even when you have treats, he should keep his head and neck in line with his body instead of turning toward you. Turning his head toward you won't be rewarded; a "tidy" front-facing nose is what will get him a click and a treat. The role of a physical barrier is especially important for this exercise so that you don't have to push the horse away.

"Protective Contact"

For a couple of these first exercises, I've told you to put a physical barrier between you and your horse—this is called "protective contact," in the professional zoo trainer world. With that barrier between you (whether it's the wall of an arena, the fence of a round pen, or the door of a stall), you won't have to keep pushing the horse away from you with your hands, which should instead be associated with giving rewards—and you also avoid feeling frustrated and annoyed by having to avoid his attempts to take rewards for himself. If he tries to reach straight for your treat bag from the other side of the barrier, just take a step or two back, and you'll be out of reach. After a few withdrawals on your part, he'll understand that there's no point in reaching for you; you'll approach him when it's time for him to get a reward. You're also safe from your horse interrupting the exercise to ask you for a scratch—during these exercises, you should try to avoid any actions or gestures that don't have to do with the skills you're

What You'll Need
- The clicker (if you don't have another signal) and a bag;
- Food rewards;
- A space that physically separates you from the horse (a stall, a fence).

What You're Practicing
- Extending your arm to give rewards;
- Ignoring unwanted behavior;
- Rewarding "good" behavior.

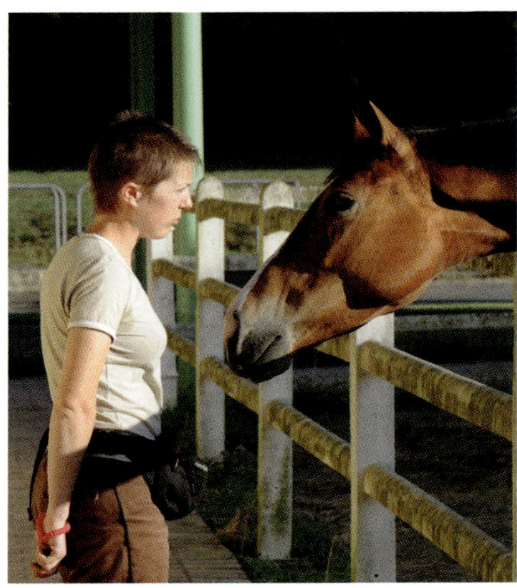

working on, because they might confuse the horse. Later on, you'll do other exercises with no barrier. But rest assured that the barrier's presence won't interfere with the training at all; some trainers who use these methods are always doing it from behind a barrier, since they're working with potentially dangerous animals (elephants, rhinoceroses, big cats), and they still get excellent results and form strong relationships with the animals they work with.

- Stand still beside the handler even though they have food;
- Wait for the food to be given instead of trying to take it.

✦ What You Do

Stand outside the horse's stall or paddock, or on the other side of whatever barrier is available to you, at the horse's shoulder or just a few steps away from him. Your hands should start out at your sides. Hold the clicker in the hand nearest to the horse (if you are standing on the left side of the horse, for example, this will be your right hand). The other hand will give him treats (if you are on the left, this will be your left hand). Watch the horse in your peripheral vision. He'll probably try to bring his nose closer to the bag of treats, or to your hands. Let him do it, without pushing him away—this behavior leads to nothing, and earns him nothing. (Make sure he can't actually get a treat on his own, or you'll reinforce looking for treats instead of waiting for them to be given!)

If he gets demanding (moving his lips against the bag or your hands), move away a little bit; if he persists, keep moving away until he can't reach you anymore. Come back as soon as he stops stretching his neck in your direction. If he starts investigating again, that's okay—be more persistent than he is, and keep moving away again. Eventually, the tiniest turn of your shoulders as if you're about to move away again will stop him. And at some point, he will move his head or neck away from you. Even if it's for some other reason, an external distraction catching his attention, take advantage of it: click, and give him a reward.

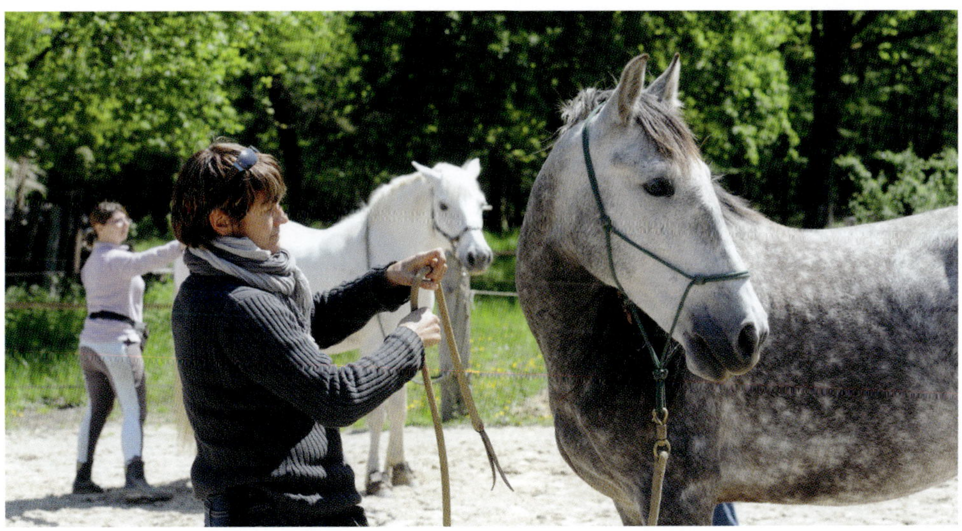

Take advantage of a distraction that gets you the behavior you want, and click!

He'll almost certainly come back to search or sniff for another treat, so you'll have to repeat your withdrawals, until at last he moves his nose away again. Click, and give him a treat. Little by little, he'll start to understand that it's the position of his head that determines when he's going to get a treat. Now it's up to you to refine the timing of your clicks until his head and neck are straight, and aligned with his body: the Statue position.

Troubleshooting: He looks toward me, and then away, and he's in the Statue position in between but doesn't hold it.
You may find that you've taught your horse not, "I do the Statue, and then get a treat," but rather, "I look around for treats, with the Statue in there somewhere, and then get a treat," because every time you've clicked and rewarded him for the correct head position, he's inevitably come back to look for more where that came from … A little ridiculous or a little annoying, depending on how you decide to feel about it. You have, probably for the first time, encouraged a "chain of behaviors": looking around, turning away, click, treat; looking around, turning away, click, treat, when what you actually want is to teach the horse to stop looking for more treats after the click and "authorized" reward arrive.

You have to break this chain, or prevent it from forming. If you're vigilant, you might spot this sequence occurring the first two or three times it happens, and then you'll be able to correct it before the horse has really learned it. To do this, start by clicking when the horse has put his nose in the right position; give him the treat, and while he's eating it, most of the time, he'll stay in the same position for at least a few seconds, with his head remaining in line with his neck and body. So—click and give him a new treat, even if his mouth is still full. You can potentially chain *this* together three or four times; you'll feel like a candy dispenser, but that's okay.

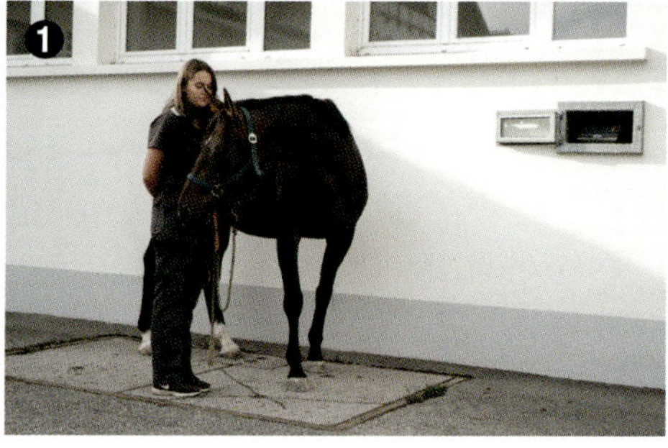

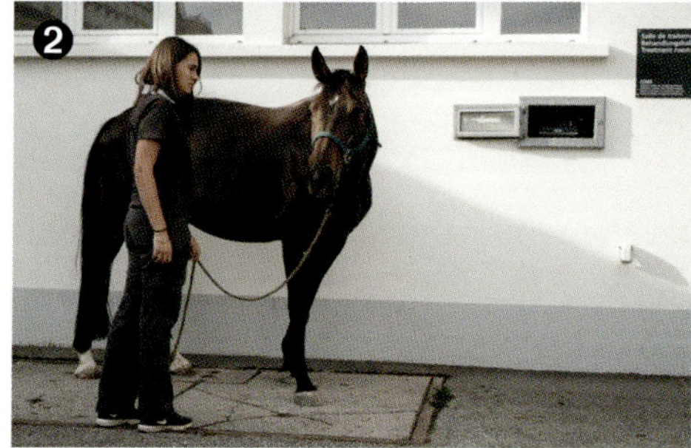

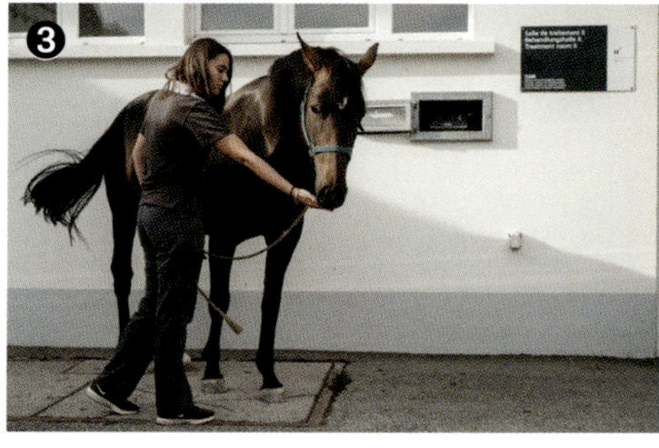

Take advantage of your horse's distraction from his environment ❷ to click and reward him ❸ even if he was searching for treats a moment before ❶.

The horse will begin to learn that there isn't any point in searching, because if he stays right where he is, the click and the treat will come to him.

Common Mistakes

- Pushing the horse away;
- Giving treats after clicking by mistake (at the wrong time);
- Having the treat in your hand during the exercise;
- Not clicking because the horse is distracted by something around him—on the contrary, take advantage of this situation and click!
- Leaving too much time between two attempts (which encourages searching);
- Practicing this exercise on only one side of the horse.

Making the Statue Last

Gradually increase the duration of the Statue: when the horse is in the right position, wait a few seconds before clicking and giving him a reward, and then a few more.

How You Move

When practicing these exercises on the left side of the horse, I told you to keep the clicker in your right hand and give rewards with the left, and vice versa on the other side. You should try the exercise both ways—not just because it's worth getting the horse you're working with used to having you on either side of him, but also because of the way our arm bones are connected to each other, and the way equine animals grip with their mouths. By following these instructions—using the hand that is farther from the horse to give him his rewards—you'll make it easier for the horse to pick up the treat with his lips instead of his teeth, because your arm bones will be naturally inclined to rotate in such a way that your hand tilts and the horse meets the surface of your palm with his upper lip as the first point of contact. If you do it the other way around—using

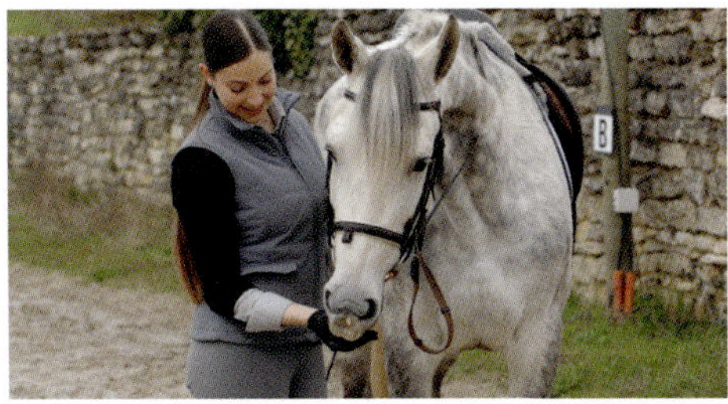

your nearer hand to give the horse his reward—your hand won't be able to tilt the same way. The horse will meet your thumb or the surface of your palm with his lower jaw first, and he'll be more likely to try to use his teeth. Equines have lots of mobility in the upper lip, which gives it great precision as a gripping tool; they are much less precise with their teeth, and are more likely to catch the edge of your hand or a finger on the way to that treat. If you follow the positioning instructions and still have trouble or find yourself dropping treats, you can hold onto the horse's noseband with one hand to slow him down, and give him the treat with the other.

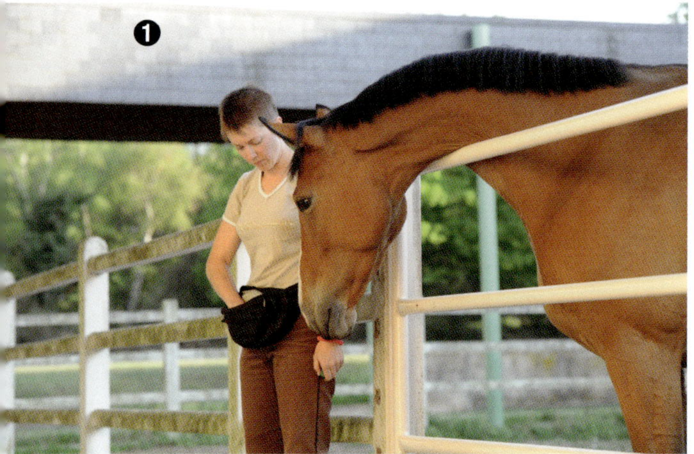

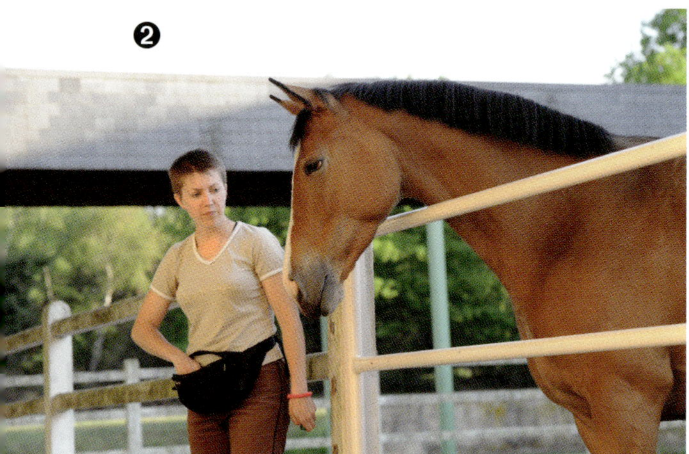

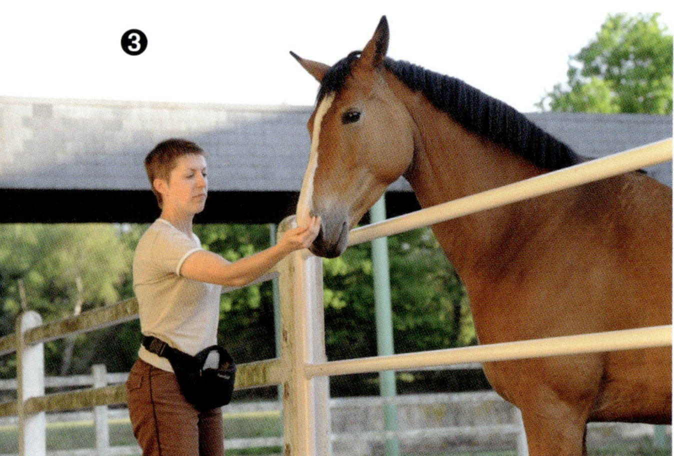

Hand in the Bag

What's the Point?

Your equine should now be pretty good at staying in Statue position when you're next to him. But you may have noticed that as soon as you reach for the bag of treats, the temptation gets too strong for him, and he turns his nose toward you again. This exercise will teach him to hold the Statue even when your hand is in the treat bag. You'll need to position yourself one more time with a barrier in between you and the horse, to keep you from disrupting the exercise because you have to push him away.

What You're Practicing

- Mastering the timing and the order in which you act;
- Extending your arm to give the horse his reward;
- Ignoring unwanted behavior;
- Encouraging "good" behavior.

What You Want the Horse to Do

Stay still even when food is being handled nearby.

✦ What You Do

This time, you will:

1. Put your hand into the treat bag, and dig around, moving your fingers through the treats to make some noise, for as long as the horse has his nose toward you;

2. Stop digging around in the bag, and then click at the moment the horse gives up on you and returns to Statue position;

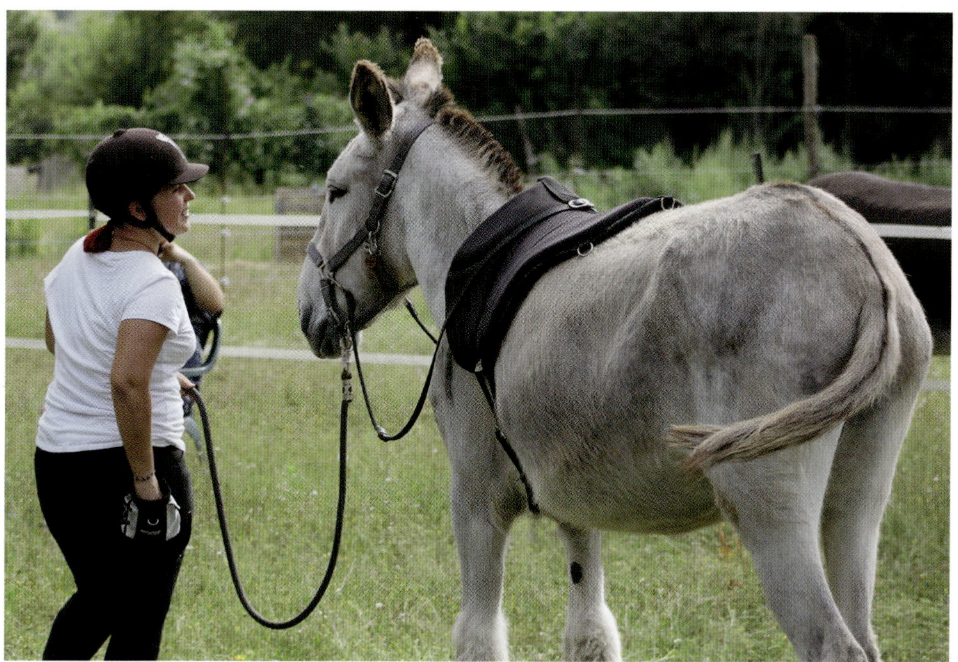

Observe how this donkey keeps her nose pointed ahead, even though her handler's hand is in the treat bag.

3. Give him a treat.

This shouldn't take too long, since your horse has already learned to do the Statue and knows his position is what controls the timing of the click, and therefore his reward. Within a few tries, he should aim his nose forward as soon as your hand is in the treat bag. If you watch his face for small movements of his nose and head, or check where he's looking even if he hasn't moved his head at all, he'll probably look like he's tempted to turn his head in your direction, but he should stay in the Statue—like he's trying to tell you you can't trick him into cracking before he gets his treat!

To refine this exercise, make sure you can move your hand towards the treat bag, not just put it inside the treat bag, and your horse won't turn toward you. If he does move his head, stop in the middle of your movement (with your hand reaching toward the treat bag, but not inside it) and wait for him to return to the correct position; then start moving again. You may need to stop more than once, but as long as he returns to the Statue each time, click and then give him a treat. Start again from the beginning, interrupting the movement in the middle if necessary, and try to make it all the way to the treat bag without rewarding the horse for returning to the Statue position—once your hand is in the treat bag, dig around again while the horse holds the Statue, and then stop, click, and give him a treat.

In this variation of Hand in the Bag, it's up to you when to stop rewarding intermediate steps and start simply interrupting your movement, waiting for the horse to resume the Statue, and then continuing until you have your hand in the bag.

Common Mistakes

- Doing this exercise on one side and not the other;
- Pushing the horse away (in this particular game, the horse is stronger and your hands are associated with food, so this is not a good time to make other kinds of movements in the horse's direction: you risk him grabbing for your fingers);
- Saying, "No!" to the horse if he does the wrong thing (this word tells him nothing about what he did wrong or what he should have done instead, so just ignore any incorrect guesses and pretend nothing happened—it's a good exercise in self-control for you!);
- Talking to the horse (this won't help him figure out what to do, and it'll take your focus away from your timing and the sequence of movements you're making).

Ask for the Statue and Maintain It

Your position next to your horse, at this point, should be a signal to him to remain still, facing straight ahead, with his head and neck aligned with his body. As you continue, you won't need to reward a Statue that lasts a few seconds anymore—you can make the horse wait longer than that to earn his treat. If you can tell your equine is struggling to concentrate, though, ask less of him, and reward him for shorter durations. Get a good, calm duration (say, 10 seconds), and then click (or signal with a word or your tongue, if you've been using those instead) and reward him. Even if you know he can do a longer Statue than that, occasional rewards for shorter durations help keep him motivated to keep trying.

This exercise is a prerequisite for any future request you want to make involving food. You'll ask for the Statue by standing at your horse's shoulder, click to acknowledge it, and reward him; then ask for it again, and this time, instead of rewarding it, you'll ask for something else, too (for example, that he stand still *and* allow you to pick up one of his front feet), and reward that. This creates a sequence (Statue, then a follow-up request, then a reward), which rewards him for giving you a Statue but at a slightly longer delay. You'll practice this in the next exercise, Switching Sides.

 — **PREPARING YOUR HORSE OR DONKEY FOR VETERINARY CARE**

Switching Sides

What's the Point?

This exercise will help you teach the horse to stay still even when people are moving around him with food. You'll gradually move away from him while he remains in Statue position. Start with a barrier between you to make this exercise easier, and then practice it in an enclosed area with a halter and lead rope, and then in a paddock with a longe line.

What You're Practicing

- Paying closer attention to your position;
- Moving around the horse with food rewards.

What You Want the Horse to Do

- Stay still when a human is moving nearby with food.

✦ What You Do

1. Ask for the Statue or do Hand in the Bag; click and give him a treat;

2. Ask for the Statue again, and this time, do not click;

3. Switch sides, turning your shoulders as you pass the horse so you take the last two steps toward the other side backwards, maintaining eye contact with the horse throughout;

4. Click and extend your arm to give him a treat;

5. Ask for the Statue again and then click and reward it, or click and reward it if the horse has

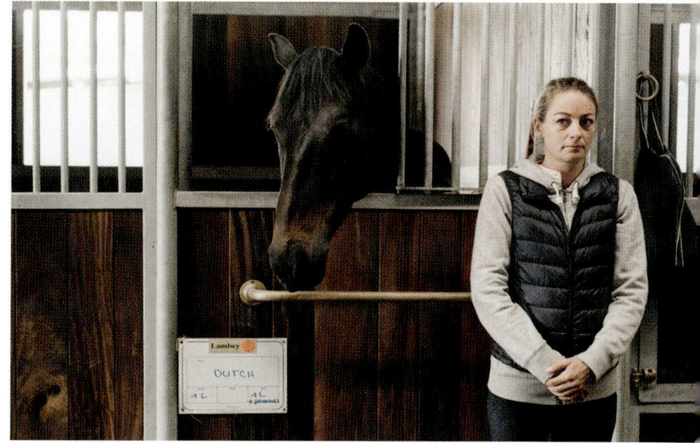

Step 2: Don't click.

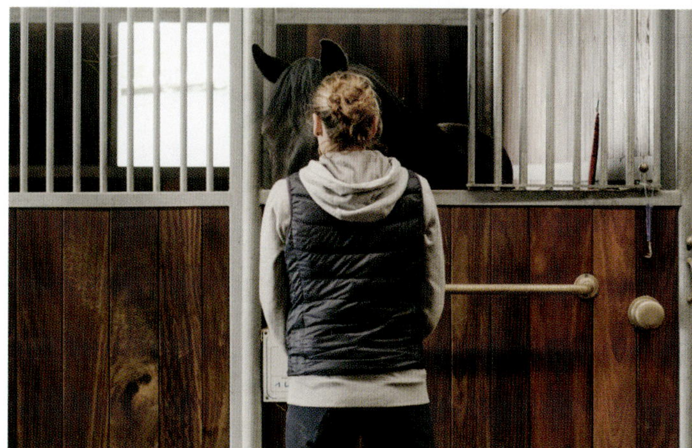

Step 3: Turn your shoulders as you pass the horse.

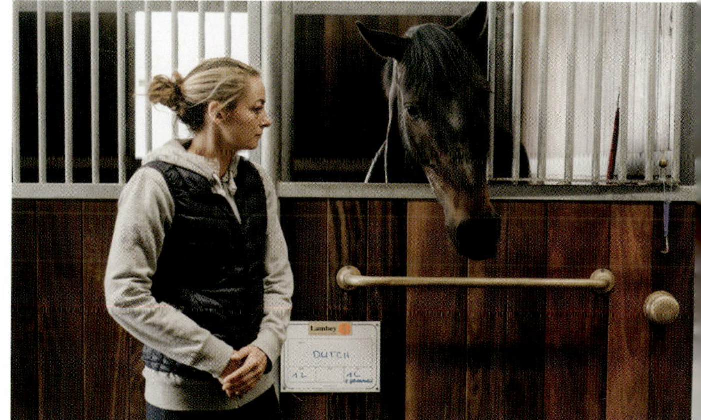

Step 3: Walk the last couple of steps backwards, maintaining eye contact.

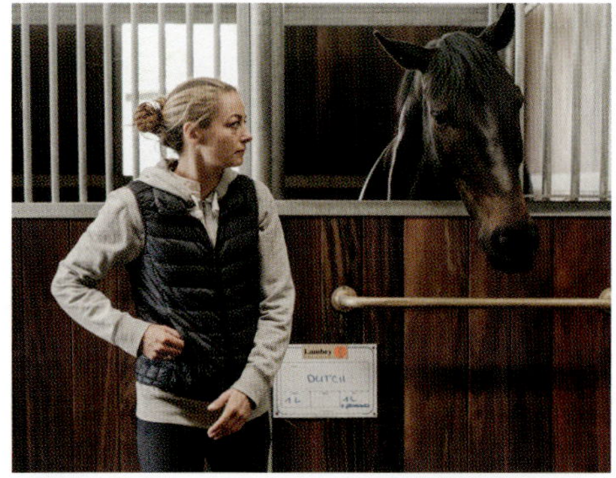

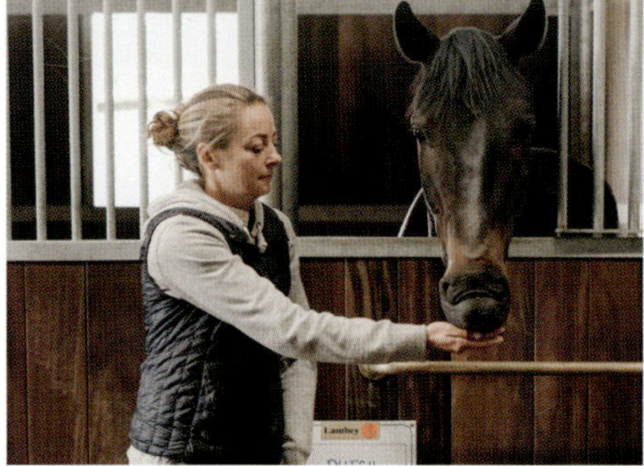

Step 4: Extend your arm to give him a treat.

continued to hold it even though you moved;

6. Ask for the Statue for two seconds, but do not click;

7. Switch back to the original side, again turning your shoulders on the way;

8. Click and reward when the horse returns to Statue position; click even before you've arrived beside him if he remains still, even if he has turned his head a little bit;

9. Repeat the Statue several more times, click and reward each of them, and then end the session.

By proceeding this way, you teach your equine that holding still (the Statue or Hand in the Bag) is the prerequisite for each of your actions. You'll be giving fewer and fewer food rewards, and creating sequences that need to be completed successfully for a reward to be given: Statue—click and reward—Statue, switch sides—click and reward—Statue—click and reward—Statue, switch sides—click and reward. As you continue practicing, you can withhold a click and reward when you Switch Sides, so the click and the food reward are not given every single time. Unpredictable reinforcement is more effective.

Once you have enough confidence in your equine's Statue to forgo a barrier, you can practice this exercise in another location to make sure it still works. If you want to take this exercise even further, you can do the same but move away instead of from side to side, either off even farther to one side or backing away from the front. You can click sometimes when you're still farther away and sometimes when you're returning to the horse and he hasn't moved, and you can also gradually increase the distance you go and the duration you want the horse to stay still.

Common Mistakes

- Giving a treat to the horse while you're still moving around him. You should separate the steps as clearly as you can: give him a treat, ask for the Statue, get it, and then move;

- Moving too quickly—if the horse seems startled or nervous, move more slowly, keeping your eyes on him.

Touch-Click

It forms the foundation for another way of teaching new behaviors besides the application and withdrawal of pressure (the principle of negative reinforcement). You'll see the benefits of being able to ask a horse to hold still while touching or being touched with all kinds of veterinary care, from palpation to blood tests, temperature-taking, and even eye care (see "Touching a Sensitive Area," "Performing an Injection," "Taking the Temperature," and "Treating the Eyes"). The term for this among trainers at zoos and parks is *targeting*: the horse learns to touch an object with part of his body, and is rewarded for it.

What's the Point?

Your equine is now used to the sound of the clicker, and associates the click with the delivery of a reward (the Click-Treat exercise). You've also gotten better at clicking at the right time. So you're ready to train your horse to understand that the delivery of the reward is actually due to his own behavior. The clicker is no longer used to tell him a reward is coming; it marks the specific moment of behavior that will result in a reward. The horse will learn that if he hears the clicker when he does something, he'll be able to repeat that behavior next time and he will get a treat.

What You're Practicing
• Setting up a learning opportunity;

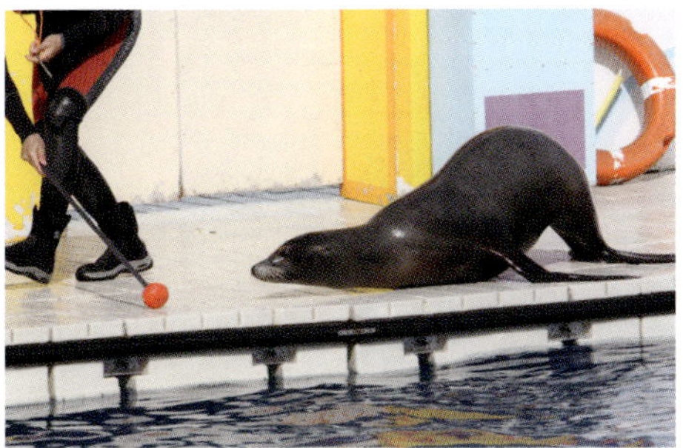

Touching a target is the foundation of many other, more complicated exercises, like moving to specific places when asked.

• Progressing through a sequence of simple objectives;
• Coordinating your movements and gestures.

What You Want the Horse to Do
• Touch an object with his nose.

✦ What You Do

An Object of Interest

First of all, you need an object—an object your horse is interested in, enough so that he wants to approach it and smell it. There is no one ideal object for this exercise; it all depends on what your equine finds interesting. You'll have to observe him carefully to figure out what else to try or what to change about the object, if it doesn't interest him at all or it makes him nervous (he moves more, backs up, refuses to approach it, or blows or snorts when you present it to him[37]).

Any object can be used for this exercise, as long as you can hold it in your hand and it doesn't pose a

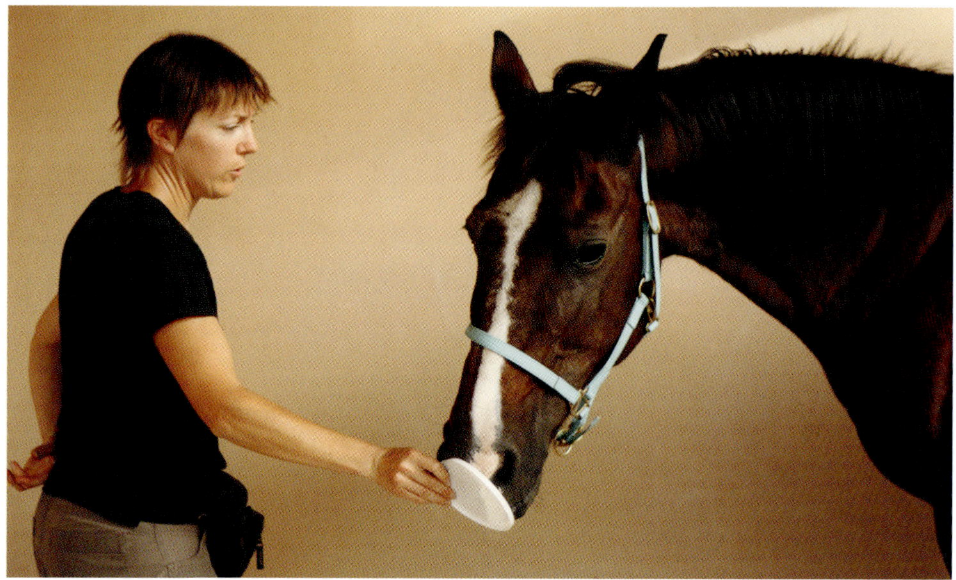

The lid of a plastic container may be a good target object—but be aware that some equines have negative associations with the color white (because of other white things like dewormer, for example), and might hesitate to touch it as a result.

danger if your horse catches it in his lips or puts his feet on it (both of which equines of all ages like to do to novel objects[38]). I don't recommend using foam objects, though, because if your horse grabs them with his teeth, they'll come apart and he might ingest pieces of them. I like to use soft plastic objects sold as toys for large dogs, which are nice and bulky, and usually easy to hold. Unfortunately, they're often expensive, and not always easy to find. In addition, some plastics have a pretty strong odor, which some equines don't like. However, they do have an advantage in their weight: they're typically light enough to be held without tiring you out, but heavy enough to be put on the ground without flying away in the first gust of wind (and potentially frightening the horse!). If you want to keep it simple, paper plates will do the trick, and so will grooming brushes or leg protection items for horses (hoof boots, leg wraps).

First Look

Start with a barrier between you and the horse. With two or three objects to hand in case one isn't interesting to the horse, present one of them. The first time, click once he's done sniffing it and give him a treat, while holding the object behind your back. The second time he sees the object, click as soon as his nose touches it, and then give him a treat.

I advise you to delay the click during the horse's first look at the object because some equines seem

 — **PREPARING YOUR HORSE OR DONKEY FOR VETERINARY CARE**

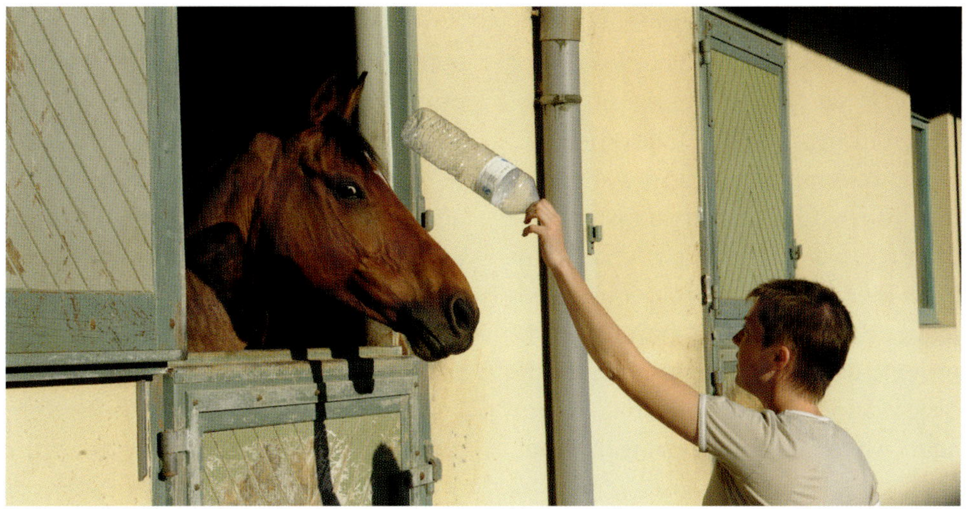

This horse is afraid of the object when it's held at this height. You have to hold it lower, where he can get a good look at it and smell it.

surprised by it, even if they were used to the clicker before, and start to visibly fear touching this unfamiliar object, which makes a noise every time they put their noses on it …

You can present your object to the horse three or four times, clicking and giving him a reward each time he touches it with his nose, even if he nips it afterward. For this part of the exercise, position the object close to the horse's nose, maybe 8 inches away. It should be up to him to close the full distance and make contact, not you!

Variations

Once the horse touches the object without hesitation at least three times in a row, you can try some variations on this exercise, either by showing him another one of your objects, or by changing position with the same object. *Don't* change both at the same time; there needs to be some continuity in the exercise, or the horse will get confused.

If you want to vary the position of the object, start by showing it to him at the same height, but hold it off to the side. Then bring it farther down, and then farther to the side, and then up toward his eye level. It's normal for equines to get uncomfortable when an object is presented to them above a certain height (typically, above their eye level), and they may even be frightened (backing up with a stiff neck, widening the eyes, minimal blinking). If this happens, be flexible; return to a step in the exercise that he does well to re-motivate and reassure him, and then try again. This is a good approach at any point if the horse no longer seems to want to touch the object.

If he still doesn't succeed with this variation, either you're increasing the difficulty of the exercise too quickly for him and you need to find a position for the object that's closer to a position where he succeeds, or it's time for both of you to take a break.

However, it may also be the case that your equine needs a faster pace than you were originally prepared for. If he seems bored, consider adopting a speedier rhythm: let him touch the object, click, reward him, hide the object; and then present it to him again while he's still chewing his treat.

No Hands!

Once your equine is at the point where he touches the object each time you present it to him, no matter its position (usually after several sessions of at least ten minutes, spread over the same day or several days), you need to check to make sure the horse understands that he needs to touch the object, not just follow the hand you're using to hold it. For horses that are still nervous about touching the object when it's above their eye level, you can skip to this variation.

Begin by taking the object and placing it in positions the horse is familiar with, allowing him to touch it, clicking, and rewarding him. After two or three successful rounds of this, place the object on the ground a few feet in front of the horse—close enough that he doesn't need to step forward to touch it, he just has to lower his head and neck. (Make sure it isn't too far away from him, which might discourage him.) If he touches it, great; click, pick up the object, and reward him, even if you're giving him a treat from a crouching position. You can keep going from here, putting the object farther and farther away from you and continuing to click and reward him for touching it.

However, it's normal for the horse to stop touching the object and come back to you when you click. It's also possible that after a few successful attempts, he'll stop touching the object and just lower his head toward it without touching it. If this happens, take the object away and then set it back on the ground to "reset." If he still doesn't touch it, take it again, offer it to him just a short distance below his nose, and then click and reward him if he touches it, and

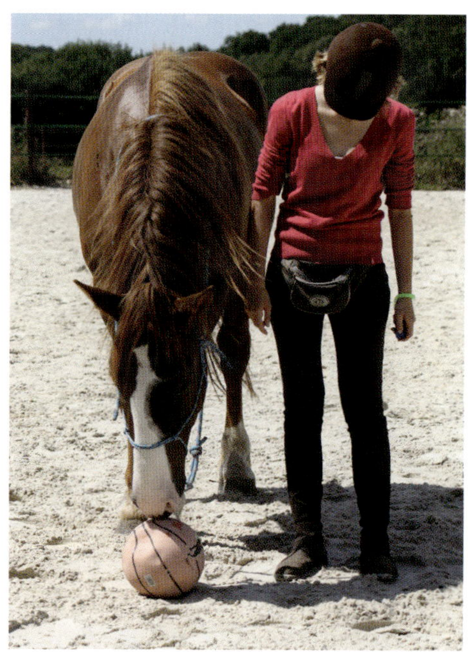

This horse proves that he knows he's supposed to touch the object, and not follow his rider's hand.

repeat that two or three times to remind him what you want him to do.

Then, try again with the object on the ground. If this still doesn't work, take a break and then begin again as explained below.

If your equine only makes a downward movement with his neck when you place the object on the ground, then you need to lower it toward the ground gradually, clicking and rewarding each step along the way. You'll find yourself crouching, with the horse touching the object you present to him quite close to the ground. Stay crouching (to one side, to avoid any stray movements of the forelegs and keep yourself safe). Pick up the object, put it down, and try bringing your hand closer to it to encourage the horse to touch it. As soon as he does, click and reward him.

Gradually, you'll move your hand away from the object, and the horse will continue to touch it even when your hand is no longer near it. You may

Leaning Is Not Encouraged

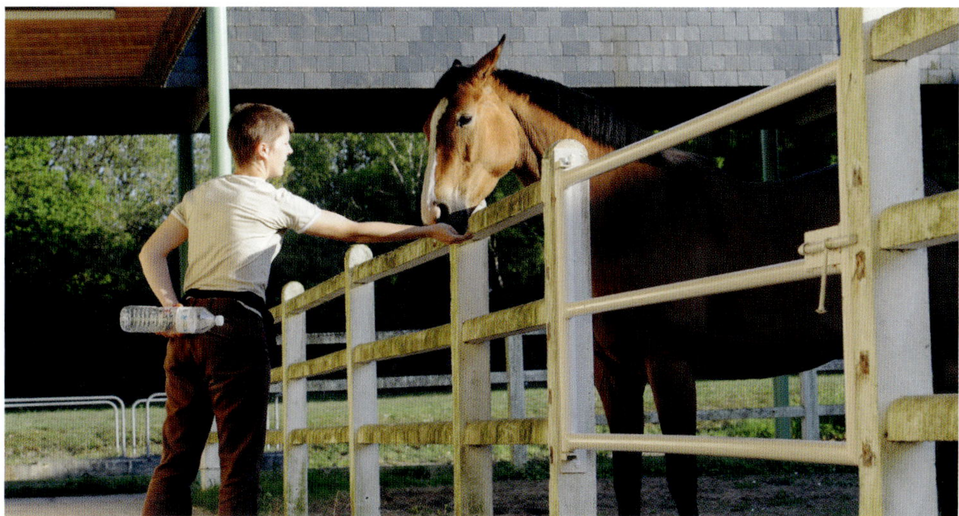

If you use a physical barrier to stop your equine from pushing into your space, he may develop a habit of leaning on that barrier—which is exactly what it's there for. As long as the horse is inclined to lean on the barrier, that means that without that limit, he would probably be leaning on you. Keep this in mind, and try to encourage him to back away a little bit when you give him a treat, or at least to "unstick" his neck and chest from the barrier when he takes the treat. Also, be careful not to encourage him to lean when you're holding an object out toward him; make sure it's close enough for him to reach it without needing to lean. If he's leaning out of habit, put the object even closer to him, to encourage him to back away a little as he touches it.

be able to stand up again, and move the object around in front of the horse. Or you may need to give the horse a few more attempts with your hand on or near the object while it's sitting on the ground, so you can click and reward him when he does the right thing and he can get a clearer idea as to what you're asking for.

Remember to take the object away after the horse has touched it, and put it behind your back before bringing it out again.

If you're still having trouble, and your equine wants to follow your hand instead of touching the object, you should take a break and return to this exercise after working a little more on Hand in the Bag and other exercises that ask the horse to be less demanding about food. This is a step that will probably be necessary at some point with every equine.

For the moment, we haven't associated any particular command with touching the object.

Equines learn in context: we present them with an object, they touch it. The next essential step is to teach them to touch when asked—and *not* to touch until asked to do so. This will help prevent them from putting their noses in everything they come across without being invited, as it will be *refraining* from poking into things that will be associated with a treat …

✦ What You Do

The order in which the exercise unfolds is also important:

1. The horse touches the object;
2. You click;
3. You hide the object;
4. You retrieve a treat;

••• Object Handling

Some advice on handling objects for this exercise: first of all, I advise you to hold your object at one end and not by the middle. Equines will spontaneously tend to direct their mouths toward your hand, since it's a hand that's been giving them their rewards. So it's important to avoid accidentally misleading them about the point of this exercise. It's about touching the object, not your hand. You also have to be careful, as you progress, to click only when the horse's nose touches the object, and not when he touches your hand while your hand is touching the object …

•••

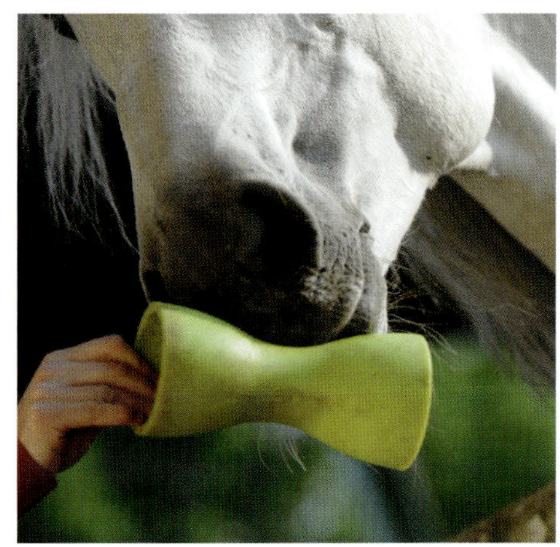

Each action needs to be very distinct. If, for example, you put your free hand in the bag before you click, you risk teaching the horse that as soon as you put your hand in the bag, he's done the right thing. You're creating an association between your hand in the bag and a reward, not the sound of the clicker and a reward, and the clicker would lose all its meaning. This kind of precision in the delineation between your actions can take time, and it can be helpful to work in pairs.

Working in Pairs

One person can stand near the horse with the object and the treats, and the other, standing at a distance, can focus on clicking at exactly the right moment. After around ten tries in each of these two roles, both partners are usually much better at keeping track of their own actions and timing when working alone. Remember to consult with each other before you begin: when one person presents the object to the horse, the partner with the clicker has to be paying attention and ready to click. If you need to discuss something, the person near the horse should move away, toward the partner with the clicker, without looking at the horse. Otherwise, you'll be asking him for his attention,[39] and he won't understand that you're reacting to something other than him.

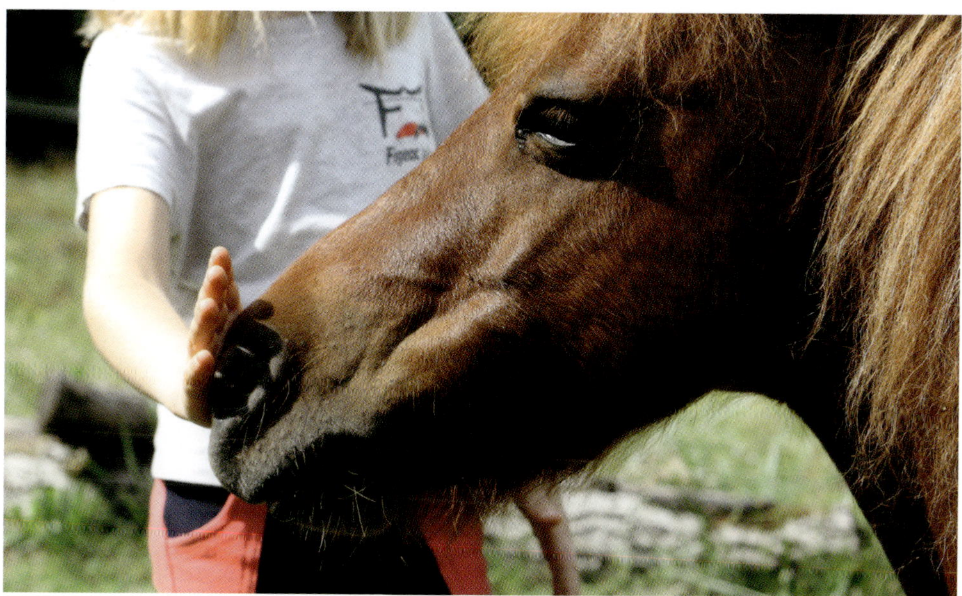

The hand will become a target eventually, but only after the animal has mastered the "politeness" exercises (Statue, Hand in the Bag, Switching Sides, and Touch-Click). Otherwise, he might try to grab your fingers. In time, though, the hand is a useful target in order to teach the "stop button" (see pages 80–84), and to train cooperation with treatment of the eyes.

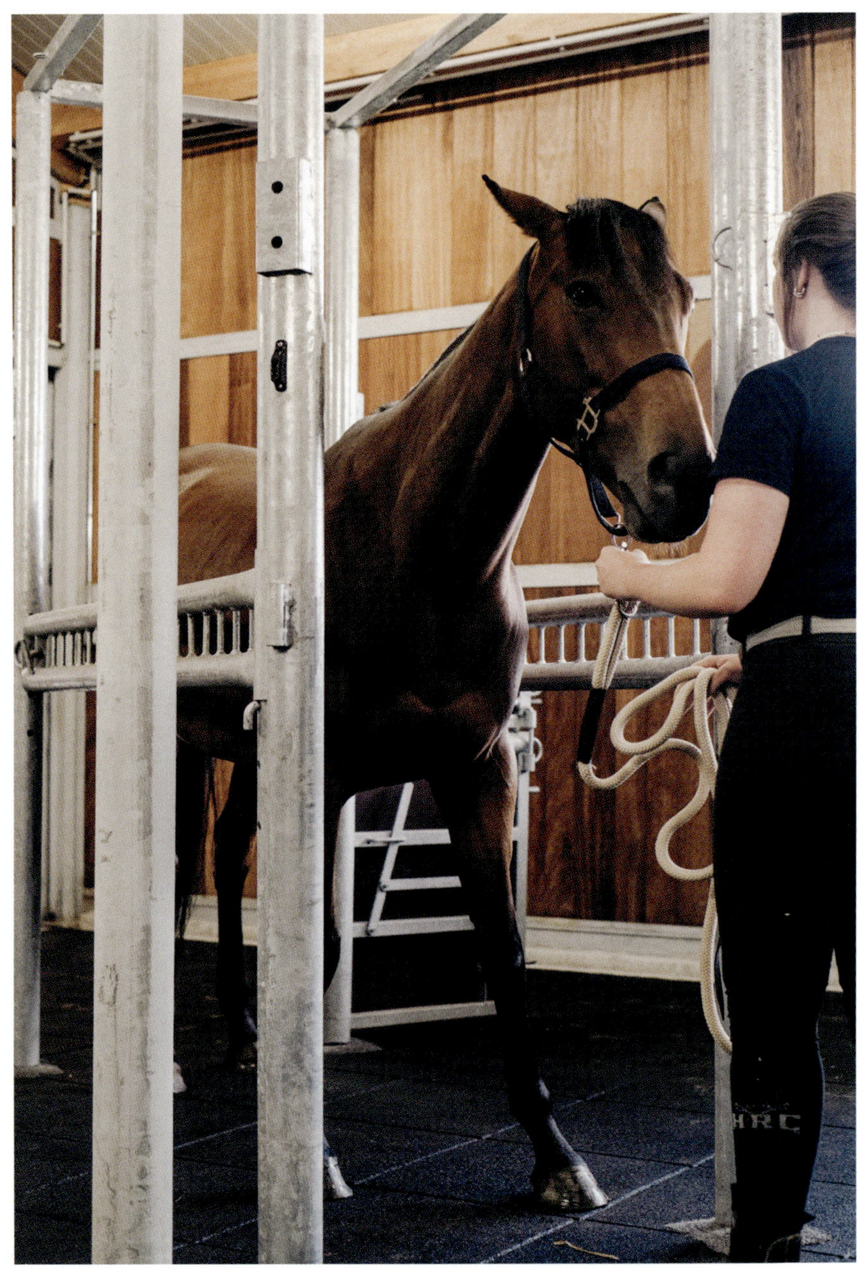

Physical restraints are easier for an equine to tolerate if he's been prepared for them. The hardest thing about horse stocks, for horses, isn't getting into them, but stopping inside of them.

 — PREPARING YOUR HORSE OR DONKEY FOR VETERINARY CARE

TRAINING FOR RESTRAINTS

Why Do It?

Restraints are intended to limit an animal's movements to allow access and intervention in a way that's safe for the operator of the restraints, other people nearby, the environment, and the animal. In this book, I'm only going to talk about restraints for an equine in a standing position, although there are also restraints of various kinds for equines who are lying down to prevent them from getting up again. Restraints are essential for certain veterinary procedures—for example, nasoesophageal cauterization (in which a probe must be inserted through a nostril in order to treat certain types of colic or esophageal obstruction). As many animals have little or no training to help them cooperate with restraints, some veterinarians are in the habit of using strong physical restraints like twitches, or chemical restraints (sedation). Even a well-trained horse, pony, or donkey can be uncooperative if he is in severe pain, or if he finds himself in an unknown place, without his friends, surrounded by humans he doesn't know. But familiarizing an equine with physical restraints will help him understand what's expected of him—that he stay still—and reduce his stress while he is restrained; it may also make some procedures possible without any restraints at all, or with minimal restraints instead of severe restraints. Training him to accept various treatments also helps with this, but it would be unrealistic and dangerous to claim restraints are never necessary.

As for chemical forms of restraint—sedation—these are usually dependent on the vet's ability to administer a successful intravenous injection. Either the animal has to cooperate out of sheer goodwill, or the vet has to take him by surprise and carry out the injection quickly. In either case, if the animal is very stressed, a high level of adrenaline in his system will make him faster to dodge contact and flee. There are also tranquilizers that can be prescribed by a vet and taken orally. These should be swallowed 30–45 minutes before the appointment begins, or put under the tongue 15–20 minutes before, depending on the type of tranquilizer. In both cases, you must pay close attention to the prescribed dosage amount and time and method of administration, for the safety of the animal and the vet alike. The effects of these oral tranquilizers vary in intensity and duration, but they can work well as a first step to make supplemental intravenous sedation possible. However, even in these cases, training your animal to accept an oral tranquilizer from you is still helpful, and you'll have a better chance of dosing him

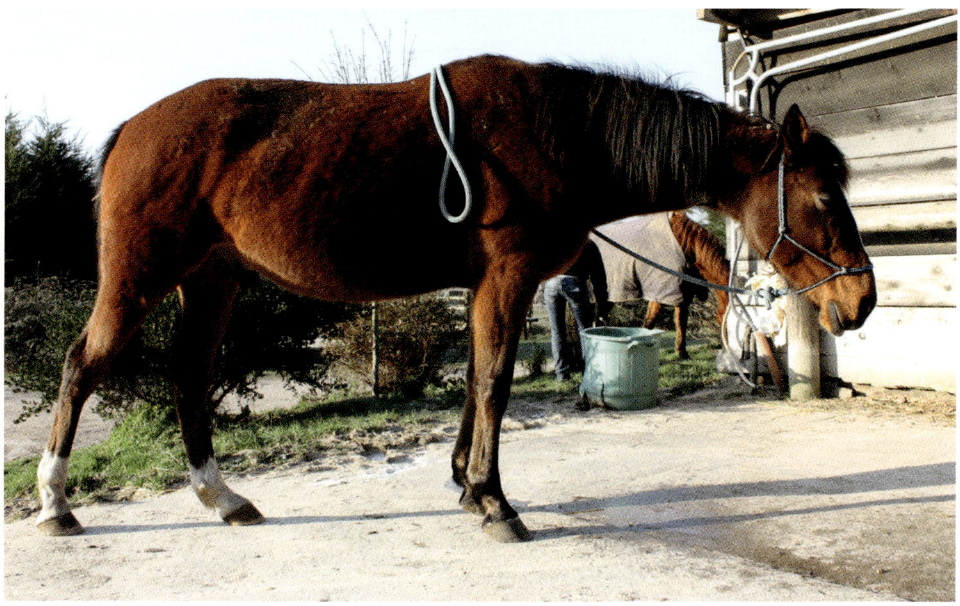

Sedation helps reduce the risks of veterinary procedures not just for people and animals, but also for potentially expensive examination equipment.

* Adrenaline is one of a category of hormones and neurotransmitters called catecholamines. Others you may have heard of include norepinephrine and dopamine. Adrenaline allows the body to prepare itself to react rapidly—for example, in order to escape from a threat—by raising a human's or animal's heart rate.

 — **PREPARING YOUR HORSE OR DONKEY FOR VETERINARY CARE**

correctly. Pain medication can also help to calm an agitated equine.

Analgesics (painkillers), if it is possible for your vet to administer them (again, either by injection or orally), also qualify as a kind of chemical restraint[40] for this reason. But even if these chemical restraints are an option, remember: if your equine is stressed, it will be much harder to sedate him effectively. So training him for these situations is still a good idea!

Also, remember that what is often taken for impatience in equines ("He's fed up with all of this!") is more likely to be a sign of fatigue or pain.[41] Increasing the degree of restraint your animal is subject to and trying to speed up to complete procedures more quickly will usually only make him more stressed or more

● ● ●

Bad Idea

Some people worry that by releasing the animal from restraint when he shows signs of impatience, they're teaching him to be less cooperative at other times (because he's learned how to make them let him go). From experience, I can assure you that this is not the case. If you're in a situation where the animal is initially cooperating with you, and over time, that cooperation wanes, that's because he's expressing fatigue, pain, or fear, and you have to prove to him that you'll respond to those concerns. No matter what you're doing, whether you're using a twitch, picking up a foreleg, or holding his mouth open with a dental speculum, if the animal grows restless, *take a break*. It will save time and reduce frustration—for both of you.

● ● ●

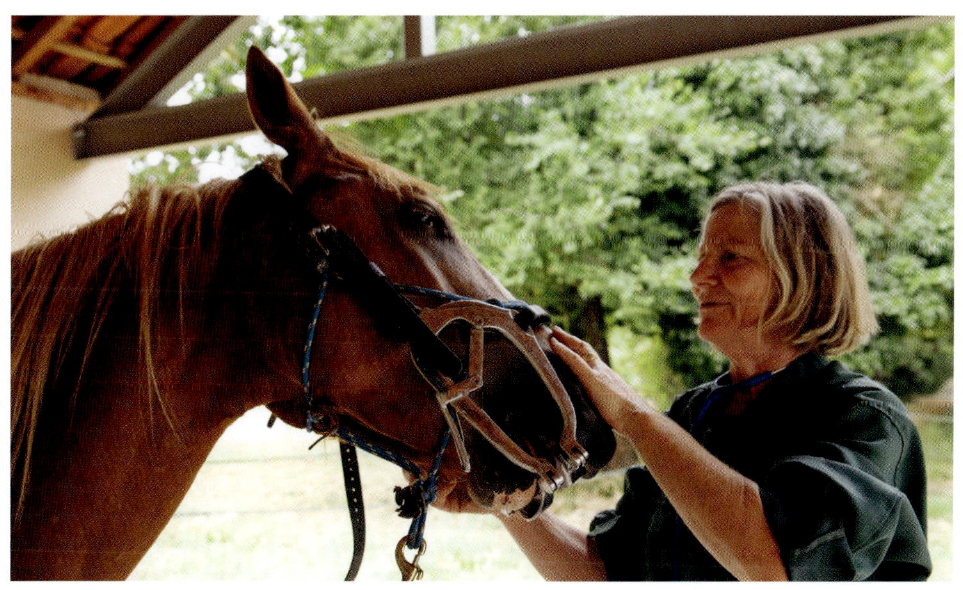

uncomfortable. Review the signs of impatience on page 25; if you notice them, it's time to take a break and release the animal from any physical restraints for a little while.

If you don't do this, you're risking the animal feeling he has to escalate to more intense behaviors that are more dangerous—kicking, rearing, fleeing, jumping, and so on. If the medical situation requires that you continue without releasing him until you're finished, this is a point at which sedation is a good idea.

The methods of physical restraint that will be discussed here vary in their intensity; some are not very restrictive and are intended to ensure the safety of people around the animal (grasping the halter, holding a foreleg, guiding the animal into a stock, restraining the head of a donkey), while others are more restrictive and are intended to immobilize the animal (grasping a fold of skin or an ear, using a twitch).[42] If your equine is very well behaved, then you may not need to use any restraints at all. But if someday he's injured when you're not around, or he needs to be taken to a clinic and handled by strangers who want to stay safe while they're treating him, then restraints might be used on him anyway. So it's always a good idea to familiarize an animal with multiple kinds of restraints—and training him to cooperate in a variety of situations will make him calmer and more cooperative in general.

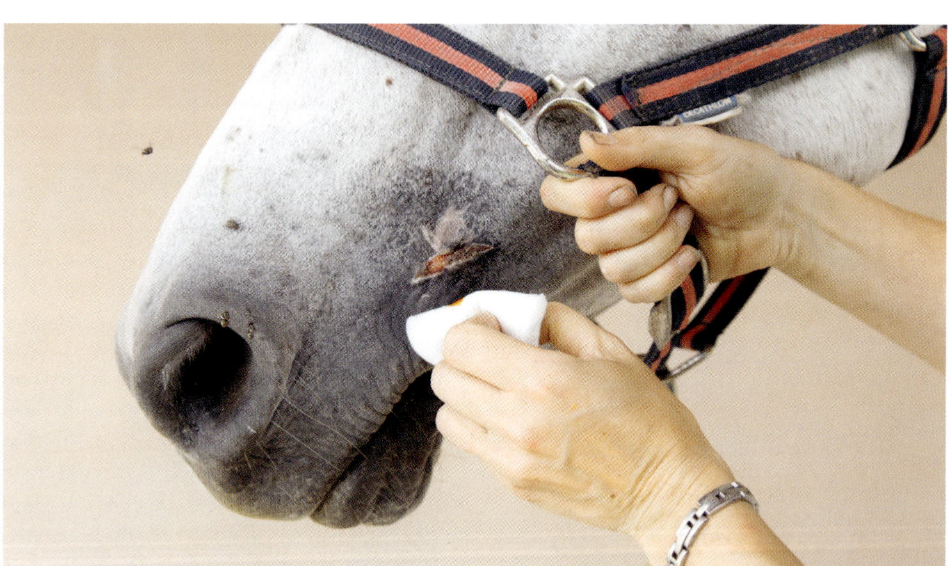

The restraint exerted here, through the grip on this horse's halter, is moderate. It's intended to limit the horse's ability to avoid contact with the compress. Head movements in this case could also occur as a reaction to the pain of the wound. So the degree of restraint should be adjusted depending on the horse's responses.

 — **PREPARING YOUR HORSE OR DONKEY FOR VETERINARY CARE**

Grasping the Halter Firmly

What's the Point?

We human beings have a tendency to grab without thinking about it. If a horse moves, our reflex is often to hold him even more tightly, trying to immobilize his head. Obviously, we do want the horse to remain still, and I'll keep repeating this: during treatment, the behavior we're trying to obtain is feet still, neck still, head still. A real marble Statue is so much easier to examine than a horse who transforms into an eel or a butterfly at the end of a lead rope. But teaching him to associate a firm grasp on his halter with positive emotions will be more constructive than subjecting him to it out of the blue, because the sensation of having his head restrained often naturally worries him and makes him want to resist by freeing his head.

What You Want the Horse to Do

- Keep his head and feet still when you grasp his halter firmly.

✦ What You Do

If your horse has previously been trained in the Statue exercise with the clicker technique (see p. 38), this exercise will be easier for both you and him. However, you can start with this exercise if you are in the middle of a veterinary intervention and the horse is reacting badly (raising his head suddenly, jerking his head upward, backing up), because working on this technique could help you avoid even more dramatic reactions as the horse escalates in his attempts to escape the pressure—for example, rearing up or striking with a foreleg.

With the horse loose but haltered, and the lead rope draped across his neck so he can't get caught in it or step on it, firmly grasp the noseband of the halter with one hand. Release and click as soon as the horse accepts your grasp and remains still. If he doesn't react, that's fine—release in this case, too! In the next moment, give a food reward. Repeat every two seconds: release-click, reward. You can gradually increase the duration between cycles of click-release-reward to around ten seconds; this is generally about the

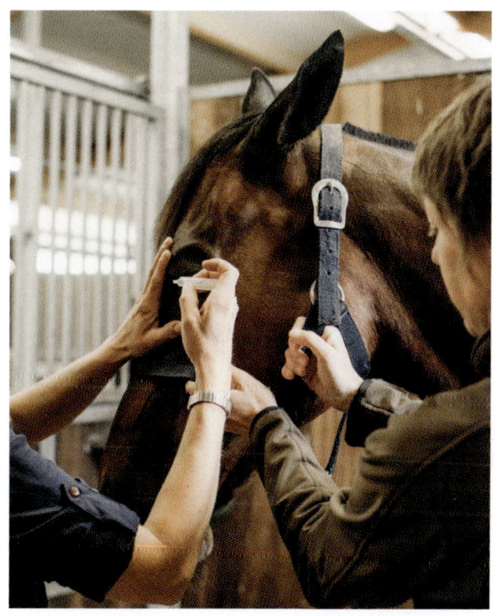

I hold the halter at the noseband and the strap between the noseband and throatlatch. The horse will hear a click and be rewarded, and at the same time, I'll release his halter and the other person will move their hands away.

same amount of time it will take a veterinarian to examine the eye, for example, or a wound on the head.

If your horse is not yet completely still on demand, letting go of the lead rope for this exercise is not going to be easy. So you can also practice this in "protected contact"—with your horse in his stall and you outside it, for example, leaving him able to pass his neck through the door or over a rope stretched across the opening, but not able to push on you or escape past you.

No matter how restless your horse is, *don't* tie him and then try to work on this exercise; it's crucial for him not to feel trapped or to decide he needs to pull away harder and then get frightened when he can't.

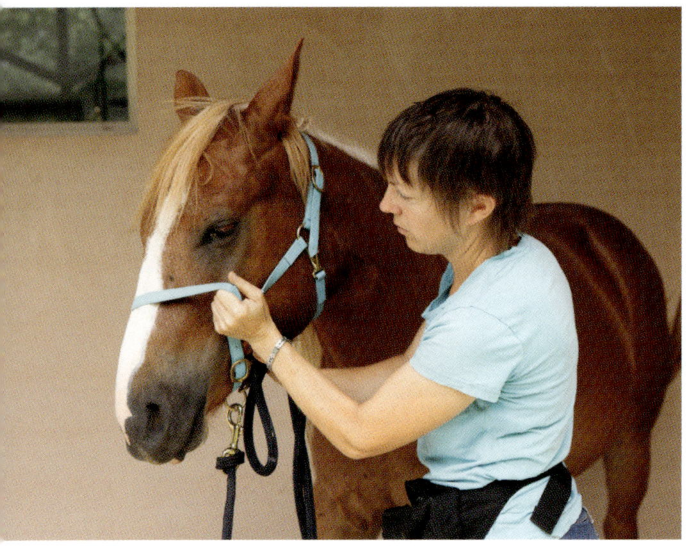

The horse lowers his head a little and lets its weight settle into the halter—but this is not the time to relax!

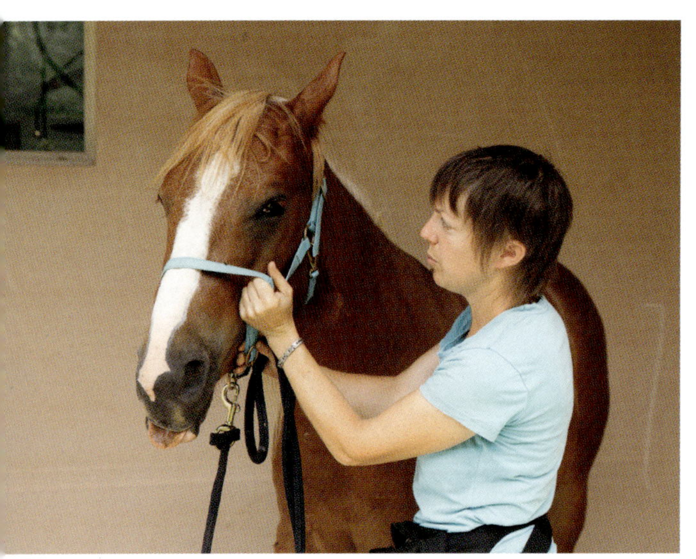

I asked the horse to straighten up, and here, he's not leaning into the halter anymore; I'll click and release him at the same time, and then reward him.

✦ Step by Step

You can train your horse this way on both his right and left sides:

1. Grasp the halter firmly for a fraction of a second;

2. As soon as the horse holds his head still, release him by lowering your arm, and click;

3. Reward him (give him a food he likes);

4. Repeat, gradually increasing the amount of time you spend holding the halter firmly, and then try holding the halter with both hands, or in a different place.

Common Mistakes

- Releasing the horse when he raises his head;
- Asking him to stand still for too long without reinforcing the behavior with a click and reward.

Using a Foreleg Hold

What's the Point?

A foreleg hold can be used when a horse is still moving too much for a complex examination or treatment—for example, an x-ray, transrectal palpation, or any other procedure that requires total immobility.

✦ What You Do

Lifting a foreleg, by itself, is a common behavior for active horses. What you want to train your horse to do is to lift a foreleg and let you hold it, in a place where he doesn't usually do that. Changing location and practicing familiar behaviors in new places is an important part of training. For example, try this in the paddock, the riding arena, the space where you normally hose him down—anywhere you would never usually clean his feet.

Be lenient, letting your horse settle into this hold for only a second or two and then rewarding him for it, even if he's very good at leaving his foot in your hand. You can gradually increase the duration, and let him set his foot back down in between. Increase the difficulty by asking your horse for his foreleg when there's another person around, since that will be the situation when the vet is present. First, just have the other person approach, and then have them retreat and click and reward the horse when they do it; then have them come increasingly close, until they reach the horse. Start out by having them touch him in one place while you're holding his foreleg; then have them move their hands all over his body, with his foreleg still in the hold.

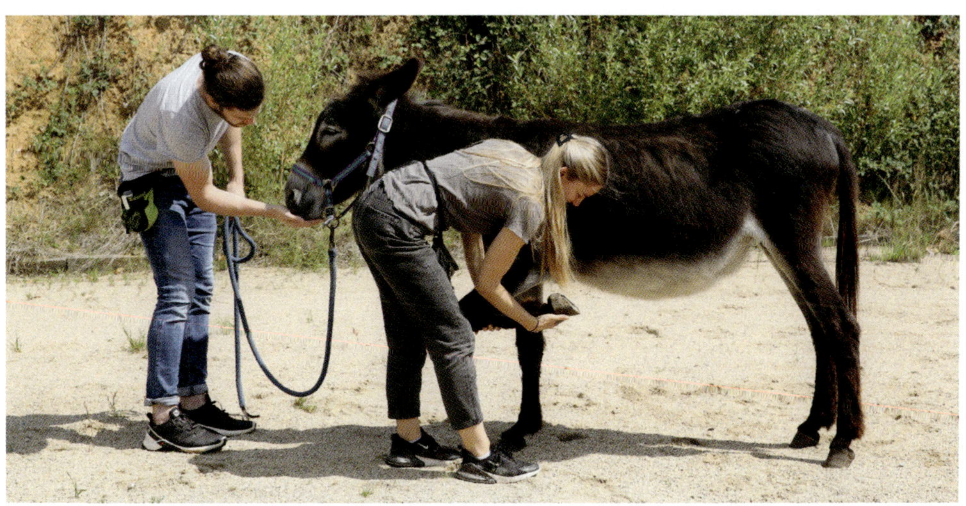

Training an animal to allow his feet to be lifted and held outside of the usual location where his feet are cleaned or he is shod—in the arena, for example—means he will be less worried about being restrained this way, should it prove necessary one day.

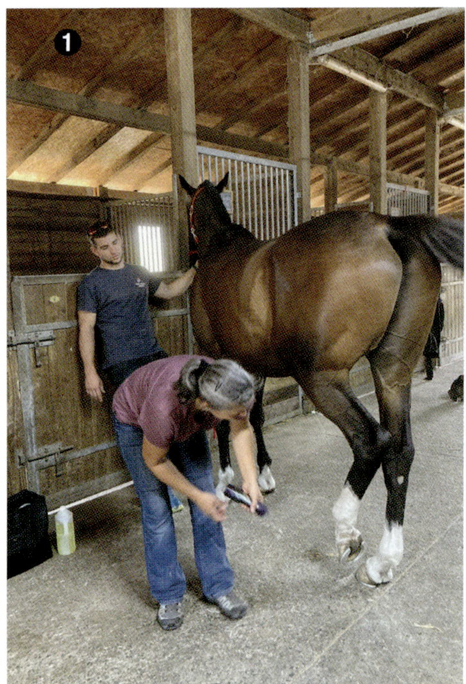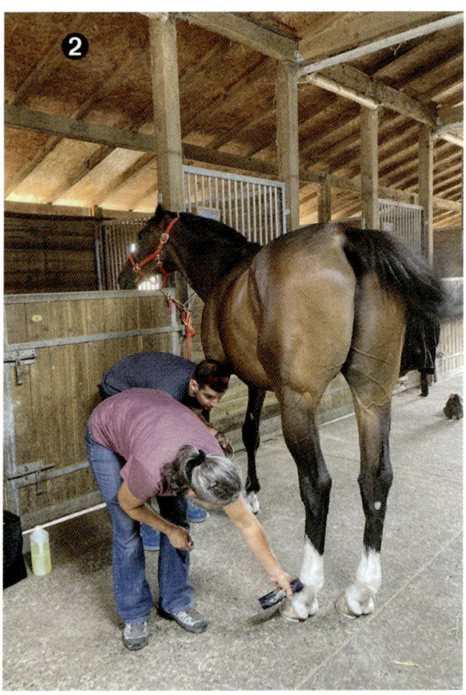

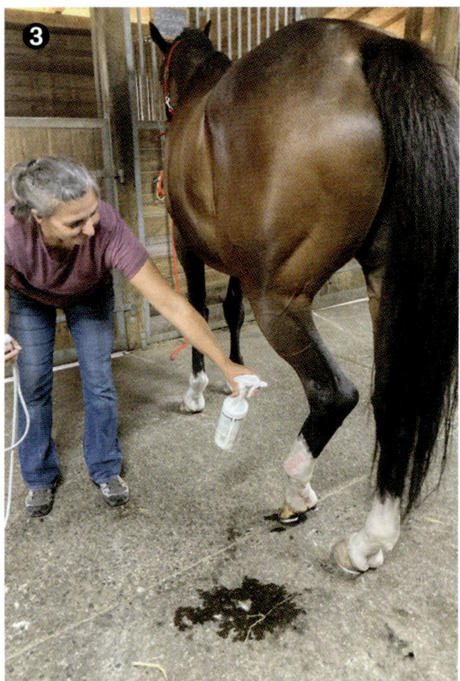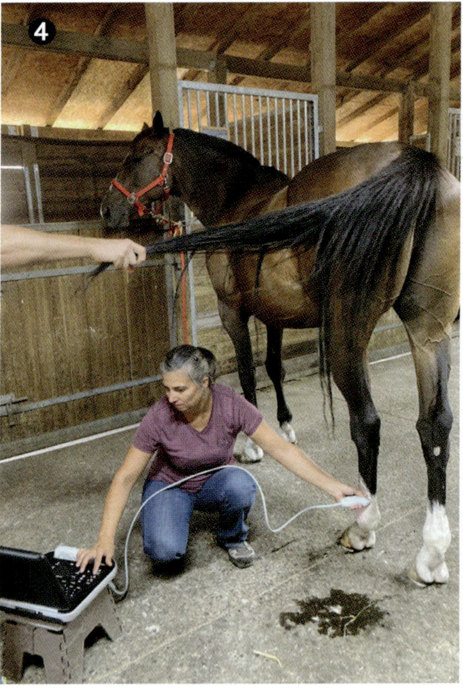

When the vet tries to clip before taking an ultrasound of the tendons in a hind leg, this horse lifts his hind foot nervously ❶. The assistant at his shoulder restrains him with a foreleg hold ❷. In reality, it turns out that it's not the presence of the nearby ultrasound probe or the clippers that were bothering him, but the flies! Fly spray is applied ❸, and a different restraint, holding the tail, allows the vet to complete the ultrasound ❹.

 —— PREPARING YOUR HORSE OR DONKEY FOR VETERINARY CARE

Using a Stock

What's the Point?

The space inside a stock is usually around the same width as a horse's body, about 32 inches (80 cm). A stock is a type of restraint that limits the horse's ability to move forward or backward, and also prevents him from turning around. It might be used for a gynecological exam, a gastrointestinal search in a case of colic, a dental exam, or even a surgical operation—for example, on the larynx. A stock like the one shown is often present at veterinary clinics and on farms. A vet can safely move behind the horse without risking a kick, thanks to the gate that closes behind the horse once he's inside the stock. Sedatives are also sometimes administered with the horse in a stock. It's a potentially useful tool to help you care for the horse—but a horse who isn't used to entering cramped spaces may get very worried about the stock.

On the plus side, unlike a trailer, a stock does have open sides, and the horse is able to see what is going on around him; in that respect, he is in some ways less confined in a stock. Training isn't *essential* for a horse that's going to be put in a stock, but remember that the more you train your horse to deal with a variety of situations he might find himself in, the less he'll panic when he encounters a situation he hasn't been trained for.

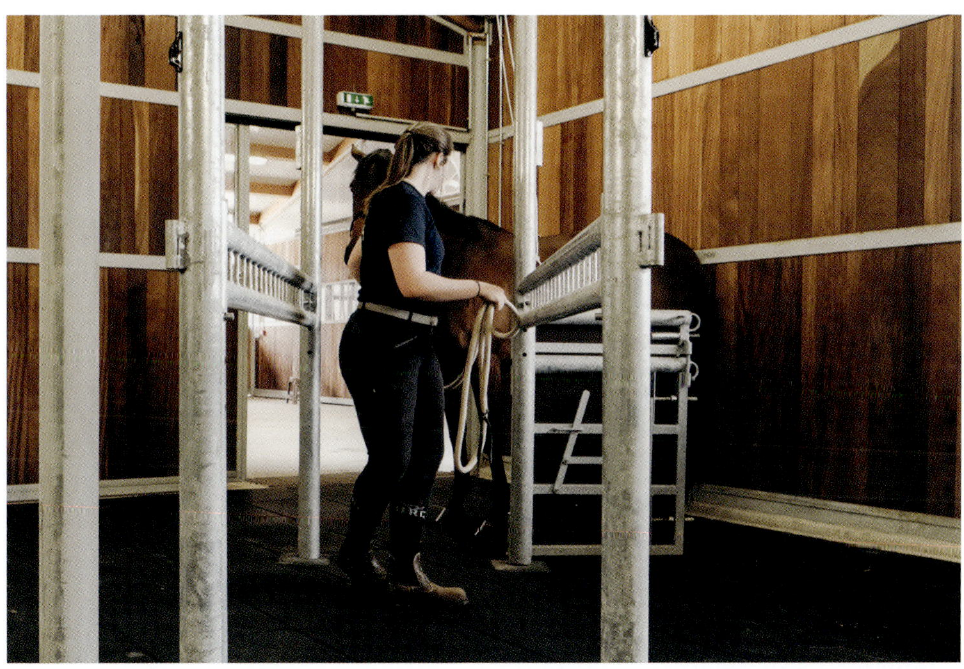

Horses don't like narrow passages. Opening the front bar on a stock—giving the horse a way out of it—often makes it easier for him to enter it.

It's also important to set up the stock in a location that isn't associated with unpleasant experiences for the horse. Otherwise, you'll have a lot more difficulty getting your horse, pony, or donkey to enter the stock, and you may not be able to get him to stop inside it—he'll just keep going and push you as hard as he has to in order to get out.

What You Want the Horse to Do

- Calmly enter the stock; stop inside; and stand still.

What You'll Need

- A wall next to which you can practice …
- … or 2 obstacle bars and 2 stanchions.

✦ What You Do

You may not have a stock you can set up whenever you want. Instead, simulate what the stock will be like for your horse. You'll be able to work on:

- Managing negative reinforcement, with pressure and the release of pressure;

- Combining negative reinforcement and positive reinforcement (marking the desired behavior, and then both releasing the pressure and giving a food reward);

- Minimizing the amount of pressure as much as possible, and maximizing positive reinforcement (using the clicker and a target).

✦ Step by Step

If you have an actual stock available, start without tying the horse. Once he's comfortable with the exercise, after several repetitions, you can tie him the way he might be tied during an actual examination, to get him used to that also.

Either way, you'll be training your horse to:

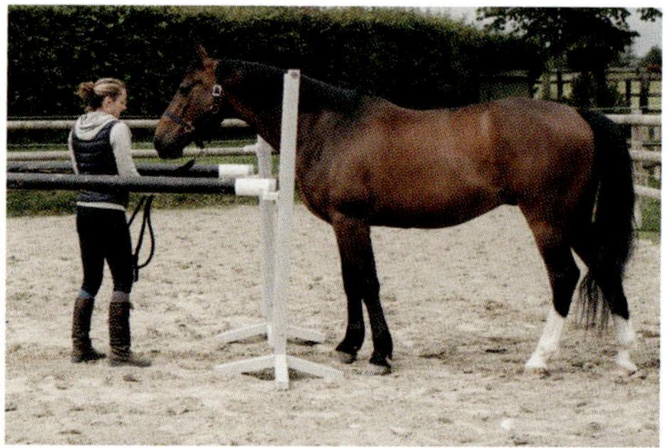

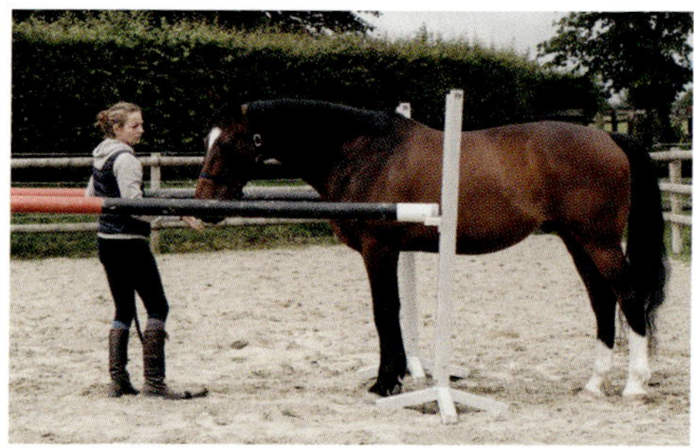

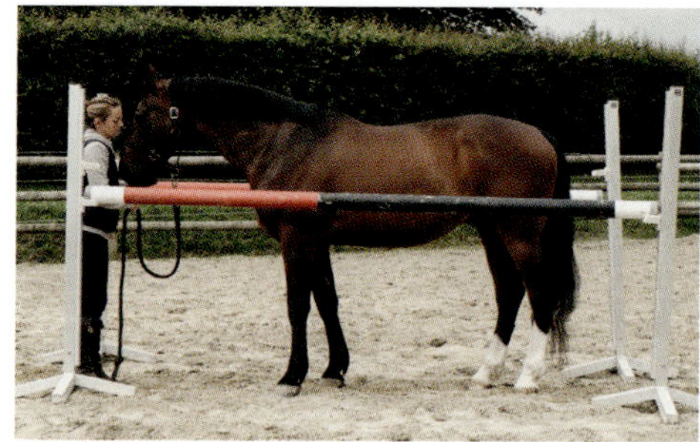

You can simulate the narrow passage of a stock with jump standards. The idea is to create a space in which you can ask the horse to walk and then come to a stop. Go step by step, rewarding each stop.

 — **PREPARING YOUR HORSE OR DONKEY FOR VETERINARY CARE**

- Move into place next to a wall;
- Move into place next to a wall and stand still there;
- Move into place next to a wall, stand still, and let himself be touched all over.

Another option that works well is to use two obstacles that you can form into a narrow corridor, into which the horse must walk, and in which he must stop when you ask him to.

The bars will be the height of the sides. With a setup like this, it'll be difficult to move the horse into it and then touch him while he's there without tangling the lead rope in the stanchions; you can stand clear and use a stick or a dressage whip to touch his back and sides instead. If you do this, *make sure before you start* that your horse isn't afraid of being touched this way outside your simulated stock.

You can also ask another person to help you by touching the horse, whether your setup is against a wall or between obstacles, while you stay at the horse's head.

Common Mistakes

- Only using a stock to prepare for invasive, uncomfortable examinations such as ultrasounds or inseminations. Your horse will learn to associate the two very quickly!

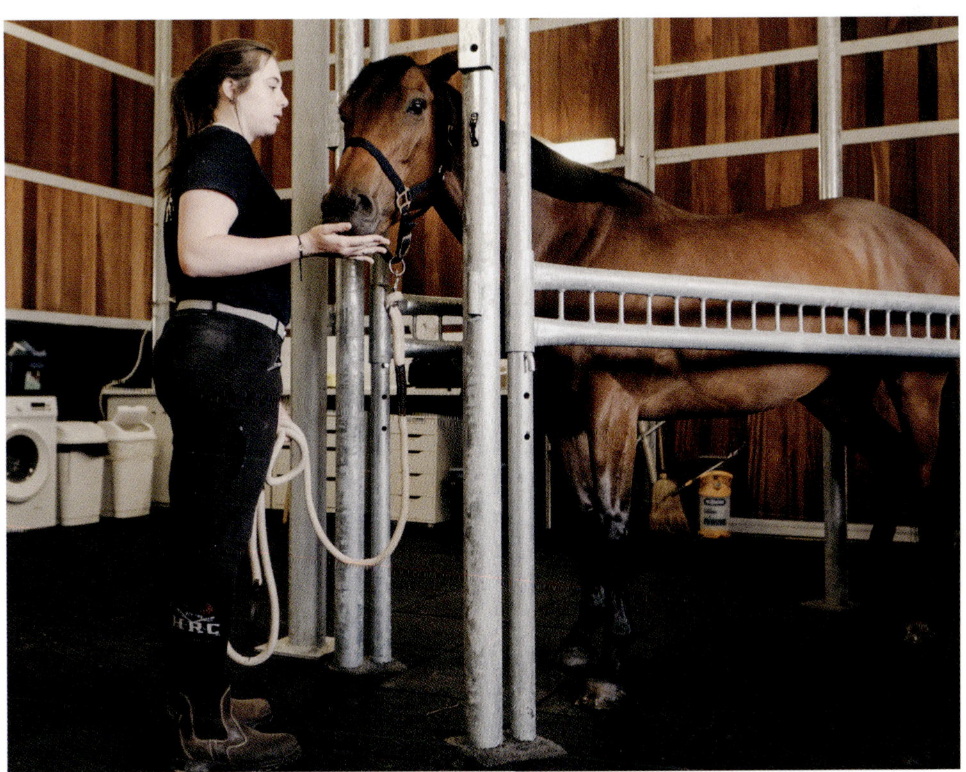

Food rewards can help the horse relax.

Taking a Fold of Skin

What's the Point?

Restraining the horse by finding and gripping a fold of skin at the neck helps reduce the horse's movement. When they're interacting with each other, playing, or mock-fighting (especially male horses, castrated or not),[43] horses will take a fold of skin on the neck of another horse between their teeth, and when this happens, you'll see a sharp reduction in the movement of the horse being held this way, and a stiffening of his neck. However, in these situations, the horse will also try to move away and turn toward the side where he's being held, in order to bite his play-fight partner in turn.[44] When you're using this technique to restrain a horse, take a fold of skin in front of his shoulder in one hand, or even both. Some veterinarians are trained to do this every time they give an injection, while others are taught to do it if the horse tries to move during an examination or treatment. Horses' reactions to this kind of restraint vary—some horses don't react at all, and others will try to "return the favor" with a bite, especially if your approach was rapid. Training your horse to understand that this is a signal to hold still will prevent problems for your vet when the time comes.

What You Want the Horse to Do

- Keep his head and feet still when someone takes hold of a fold of skin to restrain him.

✦ What You Do

You can work on this alone with a horse who's tied, making sure the horse isn't at the end of his lead so he can express his discomfort and move away if he feels the need to. You can also ask someone else to hold the horse so he's facing them, with the lead rope slack, and then you can follow the horse if he initially responds by backing up. If he tries to turn around, make sure both you and your helper are on the same side of the horse, and then bring his nose toward you both so he can't kick you.

So I personally prefer a freestanding approach, so to speak: don't tie the horse, just drape the lead rope over your forearm or over your

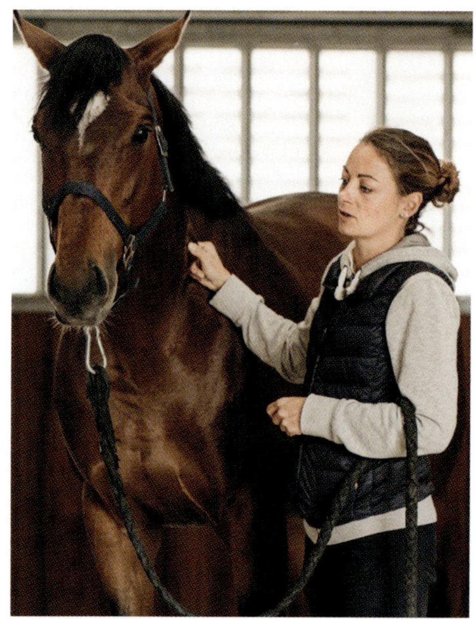

You can train your horse with this exercise by yourself —preferably, without tying him, keeping the lead rope over your arm so it doesn't trail on the ground.

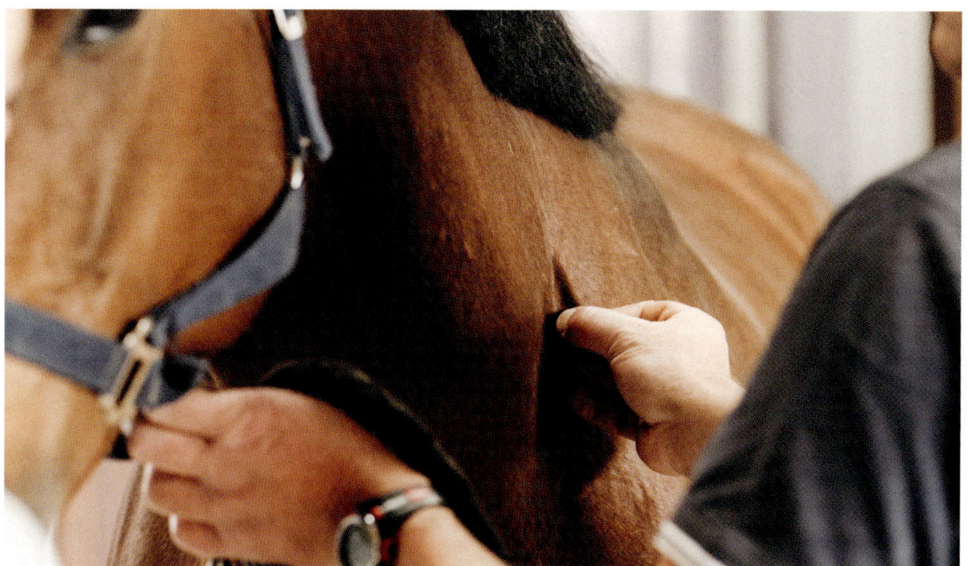

You can hold a fold of skin with your thumb and two fingers.

horse's neck. This gives your horse the freedom to move forward or backward a few steps, but you can still catch the lead rope relatively quickly. You can also take it to bring his nose toward you, if he grows panicked enough to kick out.

◆ Step by Step

1. Take a fold of skin gently between your thumb and two fingers for a fraction of a second.

2. Release it as soon as the horse is standing still (moving neither his feet nor his head), or if he hasn't moved since you took it, and click.

3. Back away.

4. Move forward again to give him his reward (a treat, food he likes).

5. Take a fold of skin more firmly, again for only a fraction of a second.

6. Release it as soon as the horse is standing still, and click.

7. Back away.

8. Move forward again to give him his reward.

9. Take a larger fold of skin firmly with one hand, yet again for only a fraction of a second.

10. Release it as soon as the horse is standing still, and click.

11. Back away.

12. Move forward again to give him his reward.

13. Repeat these steps, gradually increasing the amount of time you are keeping hold of the fold of skin.

14. Introduce another person, and have them follow the same steps, starting from the beginning with just a thumb and two fingers for a fraction of a second.

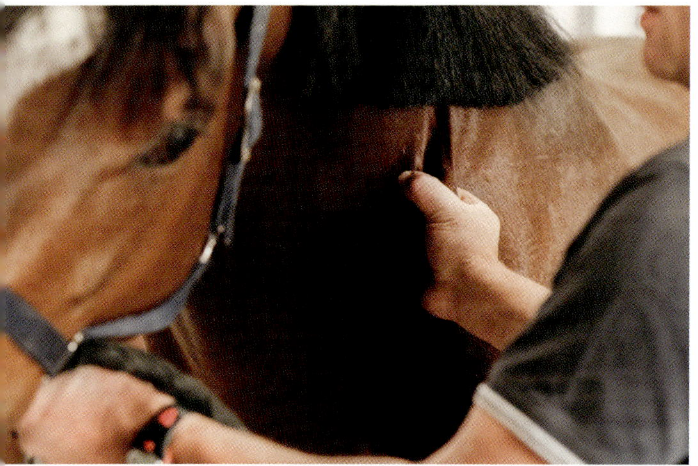

Remember that the intensity put into taking a fold of skin depends on the person doing it. Train your horse to tolerate as firm a hold as you can. Notice here that this horse is getting uncomfortable, with his head tilted toward the person restraining him.

Feel free to repeat these steps with your veterinarian present, before they restrain the horse themselves. Performing a familiar exercise with you first will reassure your horse and remind him how this form of restraint works.

Common Mistakes

- Letting go if the horse moves;
- Taking hold of the skin very suddenly;
- Holding onto the fold of skin too tightly;
- Holding onto the fold of skin too long without reinforcing the behavior with clicks and rewards.

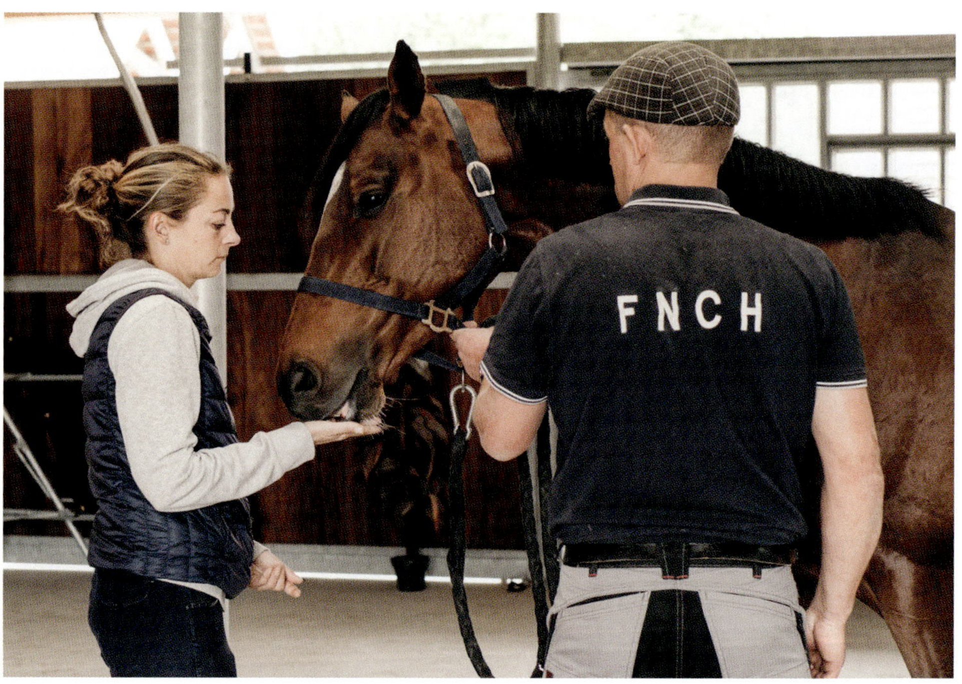

To reward cooperation, release the fold of skin at the same moment you click; the food reward should arrive only a second later.

Using a Twitch

Obviously it's best to avoid using a twitch as much as possible, if a horse has been trained to accept other forms of restraint calmly. However, as I mentioned at the beginning of this chapter, sometimes a twitch is temporarily necessary for certain kinds of procedures—intubation for an obstruction in the esophagus, to administer paraffin for certain types of colic, or for any other treatment that is necessary and urgent but so uncomfortable the horse cannot stay still on his own (transrectal palpation for colic, suturing a wound when anesthesia cannot be applied, and so on). Sometimes tranquilizers are a possibility instead of a twitch; but sometimes they're ineffective, contraindicated, or need to be avoided because a horse is required to participate in a competition for which the tranquilizers would create a positive result on a doping test. All vets have their own approach, but the use of physical and chemical restraint, along with local anesthesia if possible, is often necessary in order to treat a horse.

The use of a twitch makes many people uncomfortable. It has a spectacular effect on some horses, and causes extreme defensive reactions in other horses; both have led to categorical rejection of its use by some people, and its unconditional use by others. The specifics of any given twitch may vary, but all twitches are tools that strongly squeeze an equine's upper lip for a few minutes. Both using a twitch and removing it have caused serious accidents, and so have horses struggling to try to get it off.[45]

If a horse allows a twitch to be put onto him, he will either immediately become immobile or begin to struggle violently.

After a few minutes, sometimes horses will seem almost drowsy. To date, there have been no studies determining exactly what it is that's happening when a twitch is put onto a horse. There is no scientific evidence confirming that a twitch creates a calming effect thanks to a pressure point on the upper lip,[46] nor that it triggers a release of endorphins.[47] There is also no scientific evidence suggesting that twitches cause intense pain. The only study that has ever tried to examine the effect of a twitch had major methodological

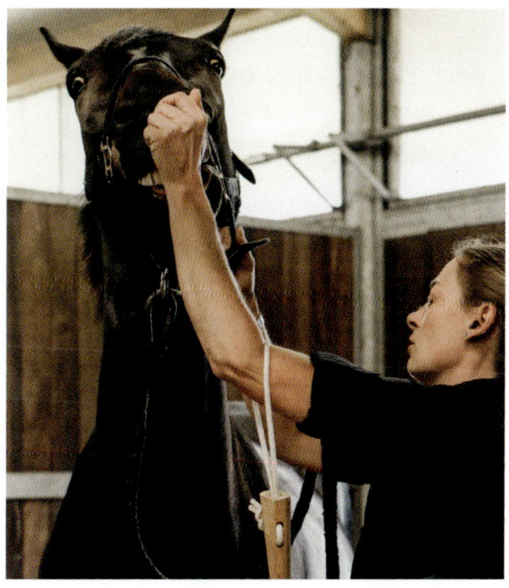

This horse is worried, and does not want to hold still to allow a twitch to be put on—he knows it's coming thanks to the grip on his lip.

problems that prevent us from drawing any firm conclusions.[48]

As for variations like using the twist on one of the horse's ears, or grabbing the ear itself and twisting it, these should be *avoided without exception.* Even if the horse does hold still while this is happening, he'll usually do whatever he can to avoid having his ear touched again afterward, sometimes for years.[49] The effect in these cases *does* appear to be the result of involuntary immobility due to extreme fear, extreme pain, or both. Horses are almost always very sensitive around their ears. My personal observations of stallions who are fighting with each other—not mock-fighting for fun, but genuinely fighting—is that when they bite each other's ears, the horse who is bitten is usually unable to do anything about it, despite extreme agitation, which definitely suggests that it's a very painful experience. So, if the use of a twitch can't be avoided, then the twitch should only ever be applied to the upper lip, and never to the ear. It also should be used for the briefest possible amount of time (10 minutes at the absolute maximum); it shouldn't be shaken or tugged on once it's in position, so if it's dislodged or coming loose, it's best to remove it completely and then put it back on rather than yank it around.[50]

If you're in a situation where a twitch is absolutely necessary, then you are facing an emergency. So if you can reduce your horse's stress and fear by training him to allow a twitch to be put onto him, you are making it easier for both of you to deal with that emergency when it comes. And training is a good way to teach your horse to allow the tip of his nose and his lip to be manipulated.

What You Want the Horse to Do

Remain still (everywhere, including the feet, the head, and the mouth) when his lip is touched or manipulated.

✦ What You Do

It's easier to practice this exercise with just you and your horse; involving another person risks them getting in your way. You can work on it in the horse's stall, or in an open space (grooming area, riding arena, longeing arena); either way, the horse should not be tied. He has to be able to raise his head, and if he's tied and feels tension when he tries to do that, he'll only raise it higher or even rear, trying to free his head from whatever is holding it down.

✦ Step by Step

Check to make sure your horse is willing to accept your hand against his head, including on his nose; if not, work on that first.

1. Touch a nostril on one side of his face, and then move down toward his upper lip, with your hand flat; click.

2. Lift your hand away; reward him.

3. Touch him again, as before, and then take his lip between your

thumb and index finger, squeezing very lightly; click.

4. Lift your hand away; reward him.

5. Touch him again, the same way. Grip his lip more firmly this time; click.

6. Release his lip, lift your hand away, and reward him.

7. Touch him again—this time, grasp the lip with both hands for a fraction of a second.

8. Release his lip, and click when the horse stops moving (or click if he remains still the whole time).

9. Reward him.

Keep going in the same general sequence, gradually increasing the duration of your grip on his lip.

In a follow-up session, you can start with these steps to remind him what you're asking for with this exercise, and then have another person do the same, repeating the first few steps with them. It'll only take a few minutes, and it'll help your horse adjust to the idea that other people may touch him there also, and that he should behave the same way for them that he does for you.

If the day should come when you can't avoid using a twitch, the step where your horse must let his lip be gripped won't pose a problem.

Common Mistakes

- Letting go when the horse moves;
- Trying to grab the horse's lip from below, in the front, where the horse can't see your hand coming, and doing it without touching his nose first.

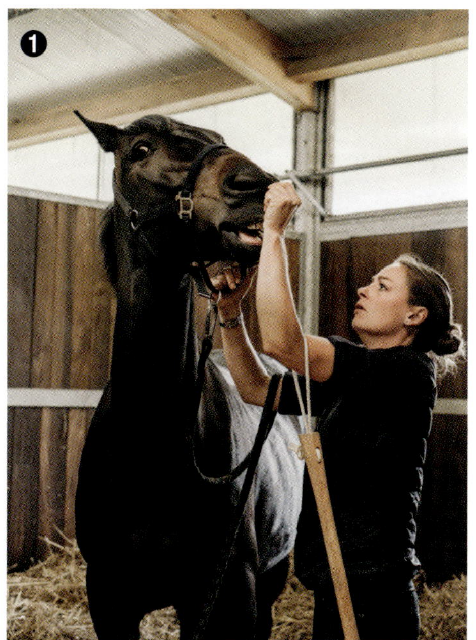

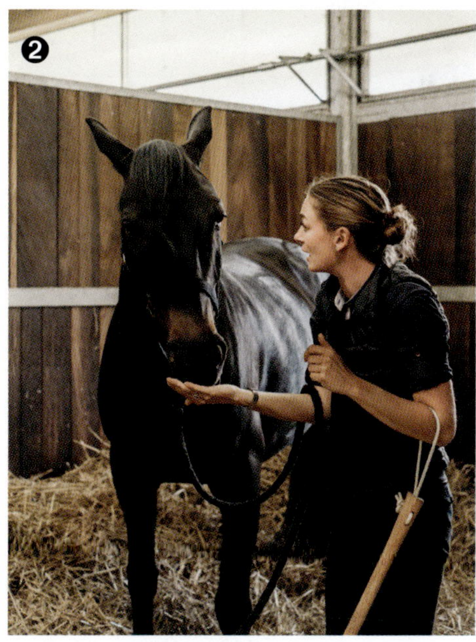

Even though this horse is clearly worried ❶, he's rewarded for his cooperation ❷.

Holding a Donkey's Head

One good way to restrain a donkey is to ask him to raise his head above the level of his withers, and then hold it firmly against your chest. The photo below shows the positioning recommended by the Donkey Sanctuary* in one of their instructional publications. You can train your donkey to cooperate with this hold.

Most of the other commonly-used restraint holds for donkeys are the same as for horses and ponies and can be trained the same way with exercises like Grasping the Halter Firmly (page 59) and Using a Foreleg Hold (page 61).

✦ Step by Step

1. Hold the head in the correct position for a second; then release it, and give the donkey a reward.

2. Repeat, gradually increasing the duration of the restraint.

* The Donkey Sanctuary is a charity located in the UK that takes in unwanted donkeys. It also gives out all kinds of information on the health and breeding of donkeys and mules. Their website is a reliable resource with plenty of scientific references: www.thedonkeysanctuary.org.uk.

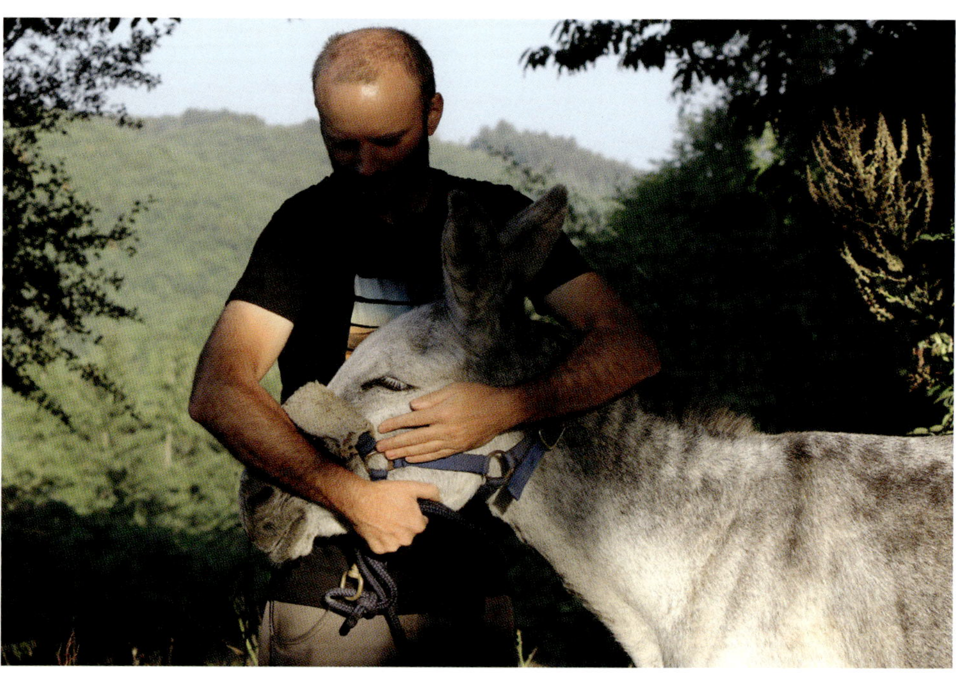

Here is the position recommended by the Donkey Sanctuary for restraining a donkey by holding his head.

 — **PREPARING YOUR HORSE OR DONKEY FOR VETERINARY CARE**

Chapter 4

TRAINING YOUR EQUINE TO ACCEPT CARE

How to Use These Exercises

All of the exercises in this chapter will be presented in essentially the same way. You'll find a training objective, linked to a particular kind of medical treatment, and an assessment of the feasibility of this training in an emergency situation; a list of any equipment you'll need for the exercise; the steps to take to achieve the training objective; and an explanation of other techniques that might help, with references to other exercises. Repeat all the steps at least twice before you move on to the next exercise. The second time through will serve as confirmation that your animal understands what he's supposed to do—if he doesn't, take your time

and run him through it again as necessary (with breaks).

Generally speaking, the point of the training presented in these exercises is for the animal to remain still and for the person to gradually approach and touch the area, approximating examination or treatment, and reward the animal's cooperation.

The method of gradually approaching the area needing examination or treatment is based on a technique called "approach-retreat" (explained in more detail on the next page). By combining this technique with clicker training, you'll vastly improve your odds of being able to carry out treatment with cooperation from your animal. Providing care isn't just about injuries! Removing ticks from under the tail, administering dewormer, cleaning the eyes … so many common tasks can be made easier with training. Treating training for care like this as important work will save you a lot of time, and it'll strengthen your relationship with your equine, too.

Touching Sensitive Places

What's the Point?

Being able to touch the horse on any part of his body is essential to allow you to make sure all is well with him on a daily basis. Your vet may also need to palpate different parts of your horse's body in order to make a diagnosis or perform a therapeutic procedure. Touch allows you to detect unusually warm areas, determine whether a swelling or lump is hard or soft, identify scabs that might otherwise be masked by hair, or, frankly, find a tick that needs to be removed

to avoid a piroplasmosis infection. There are some areas of a horse's body that are simply more sensitive than others, including the nose, the mouth, around the eyes, around the ears, between the hind legs (udders, penis, testicles), and under the tail (vulva, anus). That being said, some horses show no particular reluctance to be touched in these places, while others may be very defensive of some or all of these areas. It's part of an individual animal's personality.[52] Instead of relying on the chance that you have a horse who won't mind being touched in these places—and potentially finding out you're wrong at the worst possible moment—you might as well check, and train your horse to stay still if it turns out he needs the help.

Any area of a horse's body might suddenly prove difficult to touch if it's painful—if the horse has just gotten a shock there, or if there's an injury (a wound or lesion), or an illness or colic causing soreness, for example. Obviously, if the horse is in pain, you or a vet will want to try to determine its extent and its severity. Pain can show up at any point during a horse's lifetime, which makes it all the more important for you to be able to identify whether and where it's occurring. If the horse's pain is acute, medication (analgesics, anti-spasmodics, anti-inflammatories) can help relieve it.

What You Want the Horse to Do

• Stay still, standing square on all four feet, during touch or palpation of any part of his body.

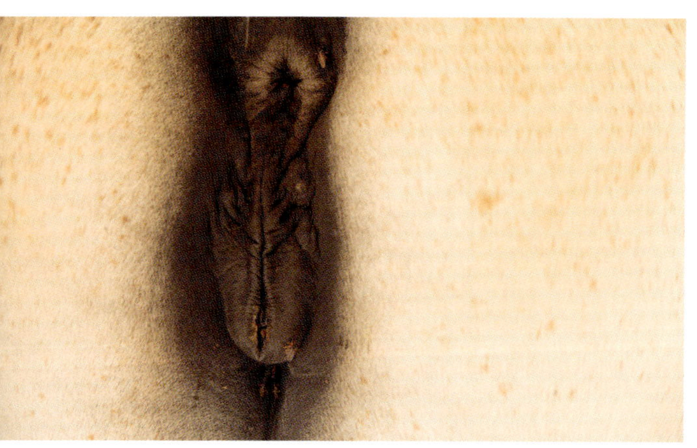

Parasites like these forest flies (Hippobosca equina) like to settle in sensitive places—here, around the anus and vulva.

Several options are available to you with this exercise, depending on how comfortable you are interpreting your horse's behavior (identifying pain, fear, or impatience, in particular—see pages 12–25). If you don't know the horse you're working with, or don't know him well, you should do this exercise with a halter and lead rope.

If you have trouble spotting signs of nervousness or discomfort in your horse, or you're worried he'll have a strong reaction (whether in the form of escape or aggression), you may prefer to work through this exercise with someone holding the horse's lead rope. Your helper should stand facing the horse, and stay slightly to one side of him—the same side you're on. If he moves, she can use the lead rope to guide the horse's head toward you both at the same time. Bringing his head around this way limits the risk of getting kicked for both of you, since the hindquarters will be aimed away from you. Your helper should keep the lead rope short but slack, forming a distinct U as long as the horse is standing still, and she should encourage his head to stay turned slightly towards the side you're working on, not away.

If you're good at handling a long lead rope (12 feet / 4 meters or more) because you do a lot of work on the ground, then you can work alone, with a halter and a longer lead rope. You still need to be careful to always encourage the horse to keep his nose toward the side of his body where you're standing.

If your horse is in a place where he feels calm, and you know you can identify any fear responses in him before they turn into actions, you can work on this exercise in a relatively large space—allowing the horse to move away if he needs to, but not too far.

You do need an enclosed space, even if it's a large one. A paddock, lungeing arena, or riding arena will work, if the horse is used to paying attention to you and staying close to you without you holding him there.

I like to work on this exercise without tying the horse, because that kind of hard limit on his ability to move will tend to make any bad reaction worse—and when I'm not in control of the position of his head, it's harder for me to avoid a kick if I need to.

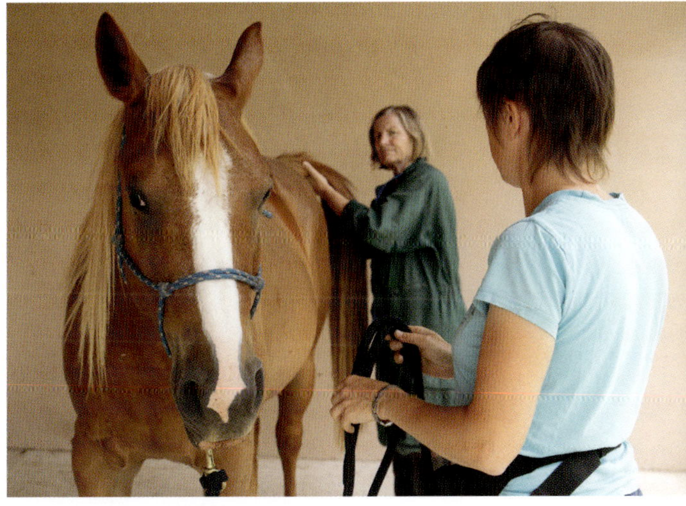

If you're working with a helper, she needs to make sure the lead rope stays short but slack, in a U shape, as long as the horse isn't moving around.

No matter which technique you're using, make absolutely sure your movements are slow, and your progress toward the area you want to touch is punctuated by stages where you're not moving toward it at all. A horse will be less reactive if you move toward him and then stand still temporarily before you lift your arms toward him, or—if you are already standing beside him—if you move your arms but keep your body still temporarily. Your touch also needs to be decisive; avoid wavering or tapping.[53] Having both hands in contact with the horse seems to make it easier for him to accept the touch, in my experience: one of them can progress following the steps of the exercise, and the other can remain still, in a neutral zone where the horse is already okay with being touched.

1. Position yourself alongside the horse, freeze in place, and then use your arms without moving your body,[54] following these steps:

2. Touch a neutral area, somewhere the horse already readily accepts touch—the shoulder, or the neck—with your hand flat.

3. When the horse stands still, take your hand away again.

4. Touch the same neutral area as before, and this time, move your flat hand in small circles, slowly advancing toward the potentially sensitive place.

5. Return to the neutral area where you started, still using small movements.

6. At the slightest reaction of the horse to your touch shifting toward the sensitive place, stop advancing; reduce the size of your circles, continuing to touch the same place.

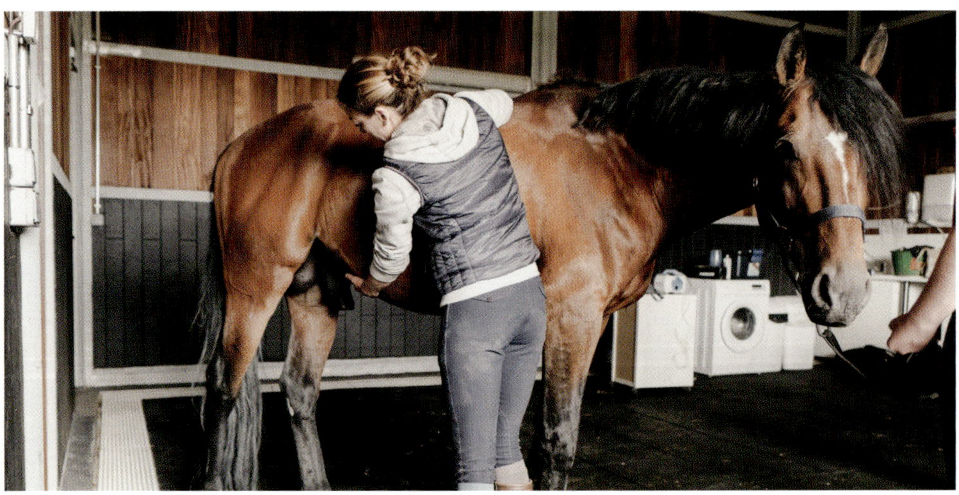

Here, the trainer places one hand on the horse's back (a neutral zone where the horse accepts touch already), keeps her feet in a fixed position, and advances her other hand slowly toward the genital area.

7. As soon as the horse's reaction stops, return from that place to the neutral area.

8. Start progressing toward the sensitive place again, in the same way as before.

9. If there's no reaction at the position that caused a reaction on step 6, go a little further.

10. In the absence of a reaction, or as soon as the next reaction stops, return to the neutral area.

11. Return to the sensitive place at least twice, for one second each time, and then return to the neutral area.

12. Increase the duration of contact the third time you return to the sensitive place, to two seconds—if there is no reaction, return to the neutral area.

If your horse does react, try backing up to a previous step before progressing again.

To add even more in-between steps to the process, for a nervous horse, try a variation: when the horse no longer shows a reaction to your touch near a sensitive place, lift your hand away entirely and step back, before picking up again with a touch to the neutral starting area. This approach is part of the approach-retreat training process for injections (see page 120) and for clipping (see page 93).

Plan on several sessions with this exercise if your horse is particularly reactive, in order to help the training stick. You'll notice an improvement over the course of these sessions, and defensive reactions should decrease and then disappear.

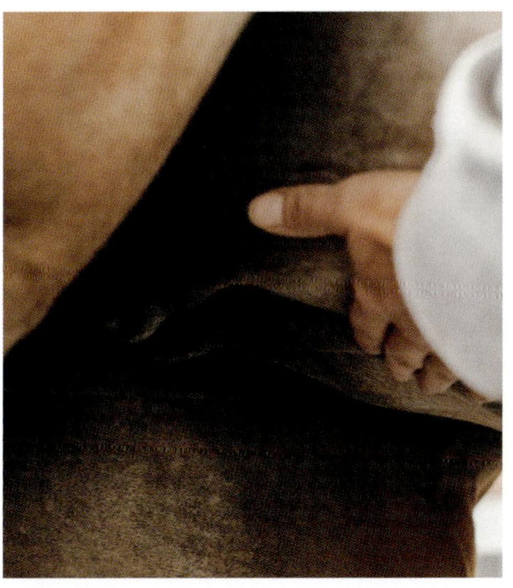

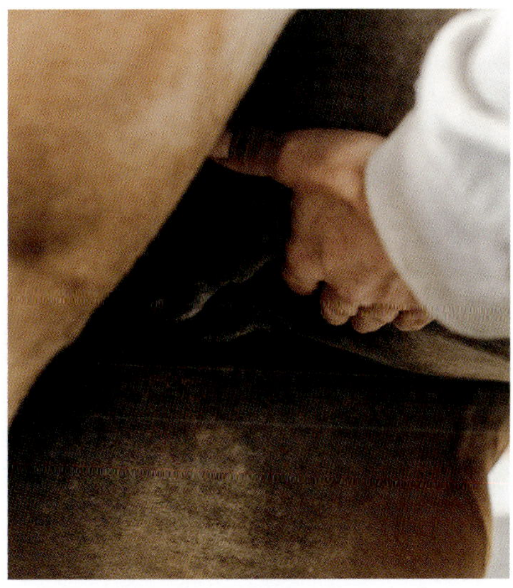

The difference in hand position between these two photographs may look very slight, but for the mare who was being touched, allowing this movement was an important step. It's the behavior of your horse that should guide the pace of your progress; split this training up into as many stages as it takes for your horse to be comfortable with what you're doing.

- Taking your hand away completely when the horse reacts to your touch approaching a sensitive place.

For horses who are extremely sensitive and prone to kicking, either to escape contact in general or to target you, use a stick that's rigid enough to create a solid touch, and use that to approach areas where the horse is reactive to touch. Many experienced trainers prefer to start out with a stick when they're working on the hindquarters (the backs of the haunches, buttocks, and hind legs). Once the horse accepts contact from the stick, they switch to using their hands. When it comes to working on these areas, the horse should always be in a halter so you can control the position of his head if necessary and bring his nose toward you to avoid a kick.

Also, when I say "rigid," I mean the stick or tool you use here needs to be something that you can hold in position without it being flexible enough to bounce when the horse moves—that would interrupt the contact you're trying to create, which only encourages the horse to move more in order to get rid of it, worsening the problem you're trying to solve.

✦ Step by Step: Approach-Retreat and the Clicker

Progress the same way as the approach-retreat by itself. However, in this case, when you lift your hand away from the sensitive area, you'll also click, take a step back, and then reward the horse with food. You can see this approach spelled out in

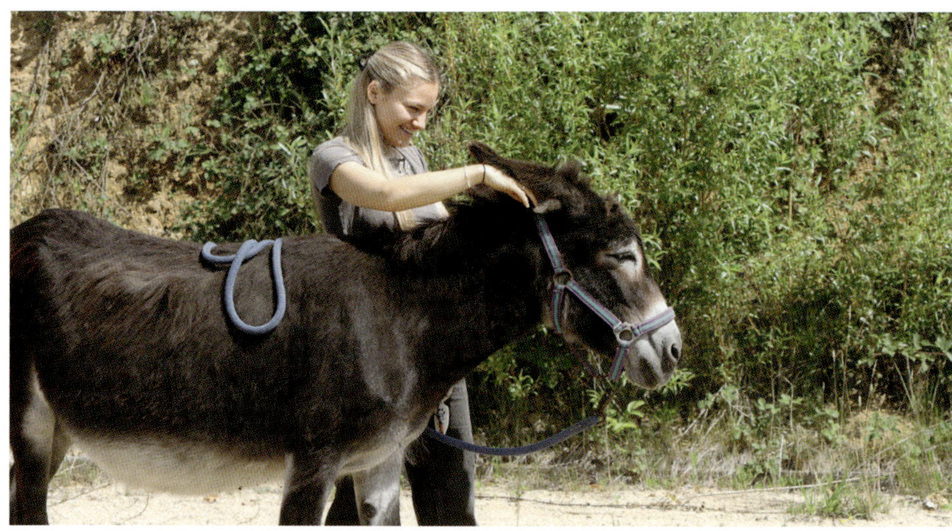

Scratching can be just as motivating as a food reward, when you're working on touching sensitive places. Donkeys in particular love to have their ears scratched, as long as you're doing it gently and gradually!

more detail in the exercise to prepare for clipping (page 93.)

1. Touch a neutral area, somewhere the horse already accepts touch readily—the shoulder, or the neck—with your hand flat.

2. Once the horse is still, click.

3. Take a step away from the horse and reward him with food.

4. Touch the same neutral area as before, and this time, move your flat hand in small circles, slowly advancing toward the potentially sensitive place.

5. If there is no reaction, or as soon as any reaction stops, lift your hand away and click.

6. Take a step away from the horse and reward him with food.

7. Repeat, moving closer and closer to the sensitive place until you are touching it.

Common Mistakes

- Lifting your hand away when the horse reacts, or when he moves his feet, head, or neck.

✦ Step by Step: The Clicker and Voluntary Contact

Another way to train a horse to accept touch at sensitive places using a clicker and rewards is by asking the horse to come into contact with your hand, using a specific part of his body. Personally, I only use this technique at the animal's head level. It can be very effective, even in cases of pain, for horses who will only briefly accept contact with approach-retreat. It takes training, of course, but once the horse has learned how it works with one part of his head, it's usually easy to teach him it applies to other parts. For example, if the horse has learned to come to you and touch your hand with his eye, he can readily learn to touch your hand with his nose, too, and keep it there while you are, say, applying ointment to a sunburn on his muzzle.

Surprisingly, the voluntary contact technique works especially well for the eyes, even in cases of acute pain like uveitis or keratitis. To practice this technique step by step, see the exercise for accepting eye care (page 137).

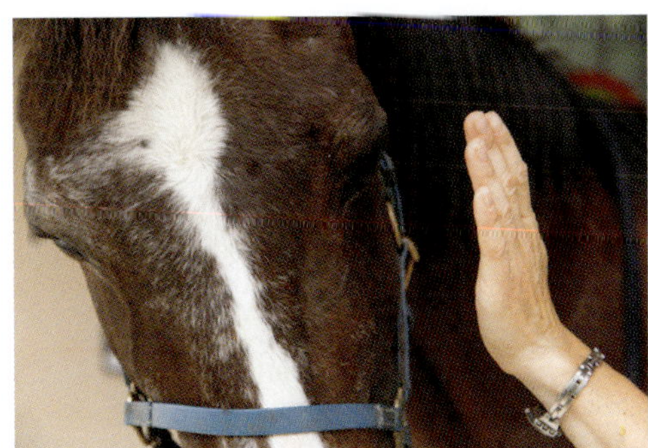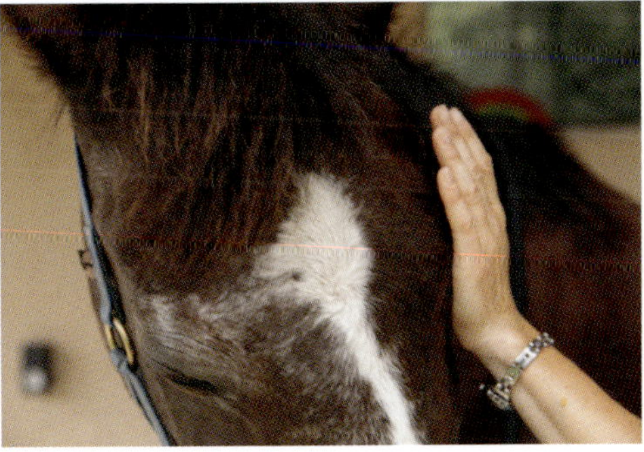

This horse has been trained to come into contact with a hand on his own, which makes caring for him easier—he'll voluntarily maintain this contact, allowing his eye to be examined or treated.

This approach involves asking the horse to hold his nose against an object, or against your hand, and stay there while someone else is moving around him. This technique is especially useful for an equine who is easily worried, since you can assess his comfort level directly: if he doesn't stay in contact with the target during treatment, but he has no problem with this exercise during training sessions, then you know he isn't comfortable, and you need to make smaller requests, for shorter durations, and reward him more. If that doesn't help, try the combination of approach-retreat and the clicker (whenever you stop touching him, click and reward). If there still is no progress on the issue, discuss it with your vet, and consider trying a tranquilizer to help keep him calm.

Before tackling this exercise, master the Touch-Click exercise (see page 47).

In the first session, your hand is the target:

1. Touch the flat of your hand to the horse's upper lip, and click.

2. Lower your hand, and give the horse a food reward.

3. Repeat several times, until you get clear contact with the horse—he should be pressing lightly into your palm.

4. Begin to delay the click by one second at a time, so your horse has to stay in contact with your hand a little longer to earn his reward. If the horse breaks off contact early, lower your hand and then present it to him again; wait just a little longer than the previous times that earned him a click, click when he succeeds, lower your hand again, and reward him.

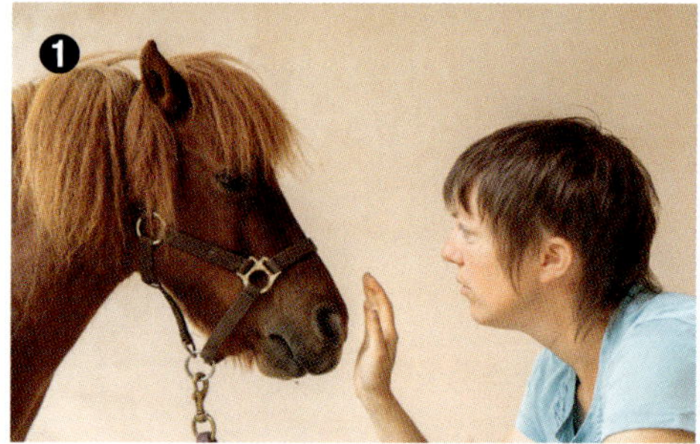

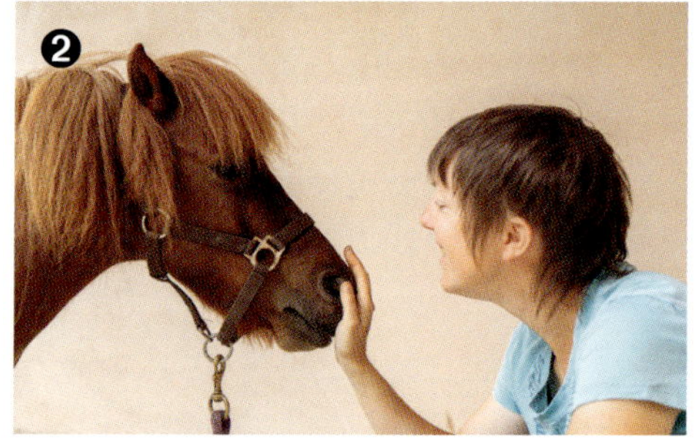

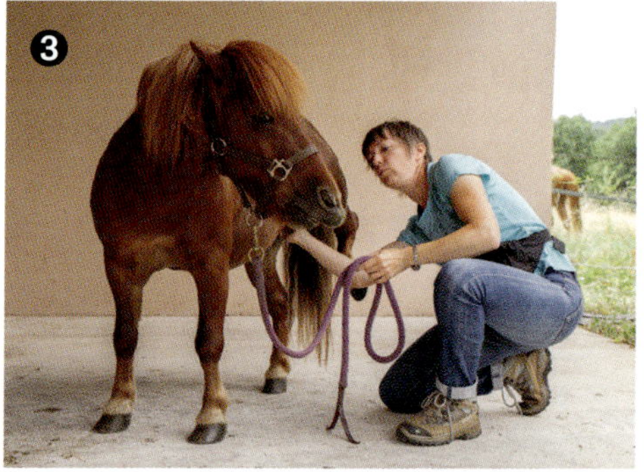

Here, the hand is the target. The pony starts out worried ❶: his neck is raised, his ears are facing backward, his mouth is contracted, and his eyes are fixed and unblinking. It's the presence of the vet nearby that's causing his concern. Nevertheless, he agrees to touch my hand ❷. I give him a scratch break during a long session, which gives him some time to enjoy himself and lowers his heart rate ❸.

5. Ask the horse to give you contact again, but for a shorter duration … and then increase the duration again by a couple of seconds.

6. Repeat once or twice more at the shorter duration … and end the session on this easy success for the horse.

During the second session, help the lesson stick and try increasing the duration some more:

1. Start with a brief contact, click, and then lower your hand and reward, just to remind the horse how this exercise works.

2. Ask the horse to stay in contact for longer periods, as you did during the first session.

During the third session, introduce distractions:

1. Make sure the horse can already maintain contact if asked.

2. Ask for contact with one hand, and move your other hand toward the horse as if to stroke his neck. If he breaks contact to look at the moving hand, lower your target hand and begin this sequence again— but this time, don't move as far with your moving hand. If he manages to stay still for this shorter movement, stop, click, lower your target hand, and reward him.

3. Repeat, still with the shorter movement, to maximize his chances of success.

4. Ask again for contact with the nose, and try to actually touch his neck

with your other hand this time; if he keeps contact throughout, click, lower both hands, and reward him.

5. Repeat, touching his neck for a longer duration before you click, lower your hands, and reward him.

6. End the session on a simple request for contact, without moving your other hand at all.

During the fourth session, introduce more distractions, proceeding in the same way—by clicking, allowing the contact to end, and rewarding the horse with food:

1. Run through the things the horse learned in previous sessions to remind him how this exercise works.

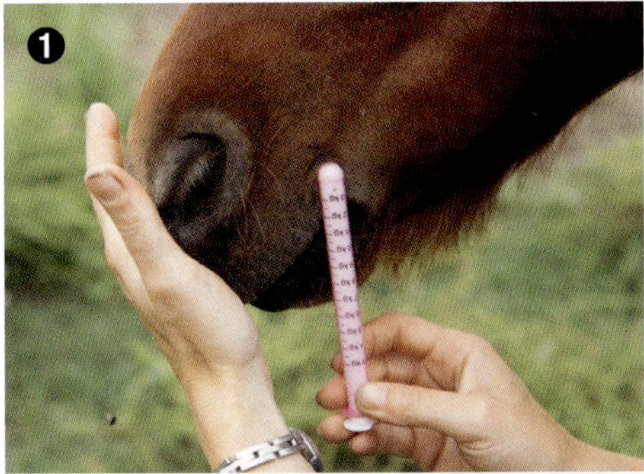

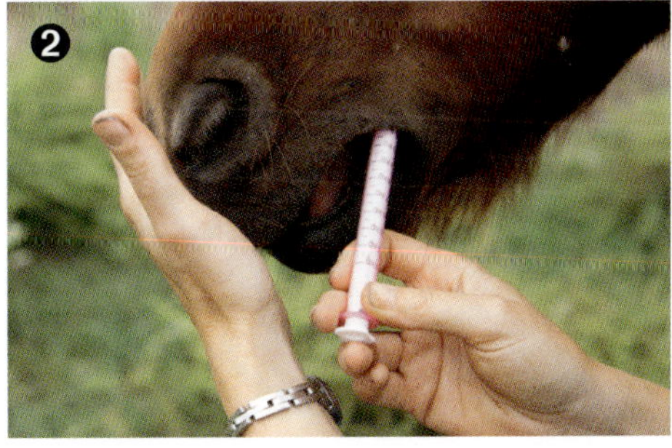

Thanks to his training, this pony maintains contact with my hand, which allows me to hold the syringe up and insert it into his mouth with his cooperation.

2. Ask for contact with your target hand, and with your free hand, lift an object toward the horse's neck. At first, this should be something familiar, and of course it should be easy to handle in one hand (a hoof pick, a leg wrap, a hoof boot, that sort of thing).

3. With his nose against the palm of your hand, touch the horse with the object.

4. Once he's let you touch him with it and you've been able to click and reward him for it, start touching him with it longer.

You can repeat this across several sessions to make sure it sinks in. The last major step is to have another person involved, while you continue to ask the horse to stay in contact with your hand.

1. Start with approach-retreat to introduce the new person into the mix. As soon as you click, your helper must stop and move back.

2. Ask the horse to touch your hand with his nose, and work on having your helper approach while he maintains contact.

3. Then progress to having him maintain contact with you while your helper is touching him.

4. Increase the duration your helper spends touching the horse.

5. Have her move her hand over the horse's body, palm flat.

6. Introduce new elements: have your helper pretend to examine the horse's eye, take a small fold of skin, or touch the horse with an object (a syringe, for example).

All of these stages should be spread out over as many sessions as necessary for the horse's peace of mind—and yours. Make sure you have the same helper available every time, if possible; if you need to swap to a new helper, be ready to back up and start with some earlier steps instead of progressing further. Remember to practice this exercise with your hand, helper, or object on both sides of the horse.

You can use an object as a target if you want to, but I would argue your hand is a better choice, for purely pragmatic reasons: that way, you

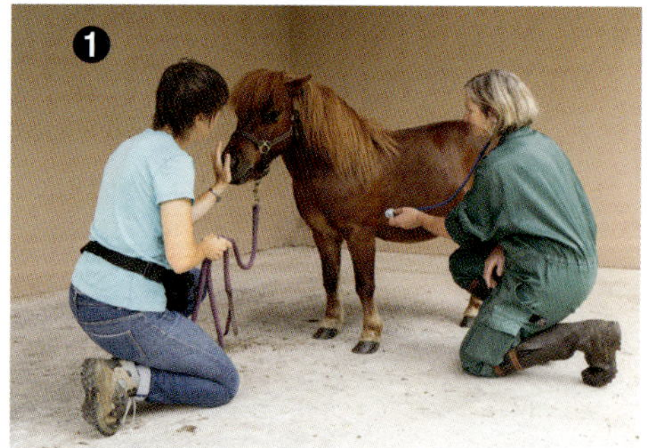
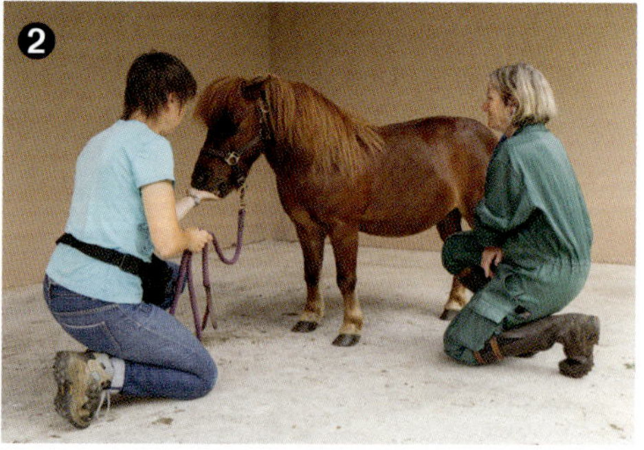

The pony stays with his nose against my hand while he's being examined. When I click my tongue, the vet immediately moves away, and I reward the pony.

 — PREPARING YOUR HORSE OR DONKEY FOR VETERINARY CARE

aren't dependent on having the object with you if you want to ask the horse to stand still, and you'll still be able to transfer this lesson to another person. Asking the horse to touch my hand also makes it easier for me to assess how he's feeling; if the contact wavers or he's hesitant about it, that's important information for me to have. I can tell when I need to encourage him with my voice, or when he might need to take a break from the procedure for a minute. I also just find this contact pleasant, and more comfortable than trying to juggle an object between me and the horse.

Common Mistakes

- Reaching out to touch the horse's nose—the whole point of this technique is for him to come to you, and offer you contact of his own free will!

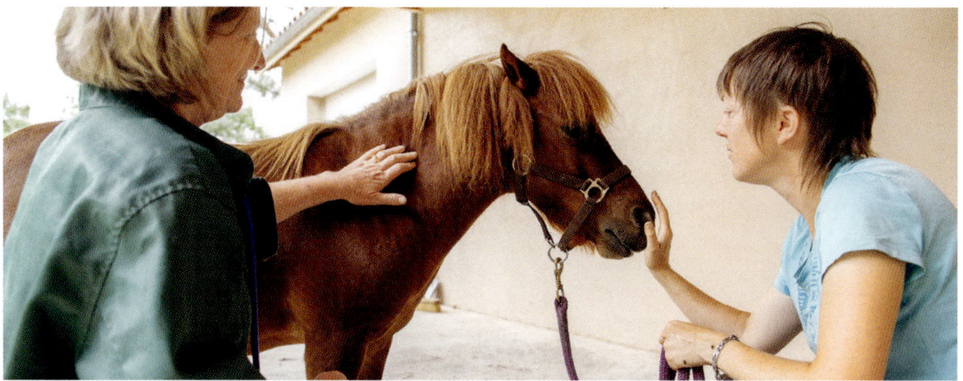

In this photo, the pony's nose is no longer touching my hand—he's letting me know he's not comfortable enough to continue maintaining contact. Now is not a good time to continue with the procedure.

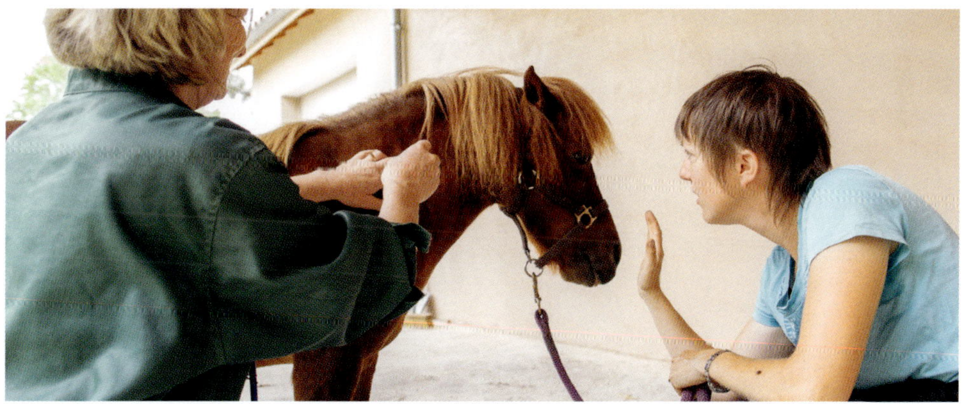

The pony breaks off the contact completely. You should stop within a few seconds of this and consider how best to continue—a mild tranquilizer might help. Here, within a few minutes of returning to earlier stages that asked less of the pony, a milestone was reached. This is a valuable form of restraint—the pony can flee or rear if he really feels like he needs to, and he won't hurt himself or me. The combined clicker and "stop button" technique is, I think, the approach that gives the most satisfaction in the long term, with plenty of notable progress along the way.

- Following the horse's nose if he starts to waver or withdraw a little bit from your hand. By doing this, you're maintaining contact when he might have broken it on his own, and robbing yourself of the chance to notice a sign that you're asking too much and he's uncomfortable.

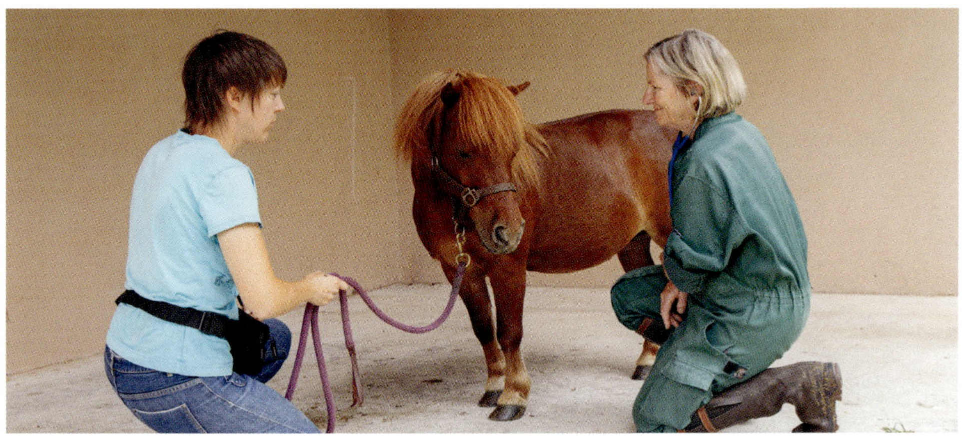

This pony had a history of fear of humans. His willingness to stand still and observe the vet here should be encouraged; it's an opportunity to reward him and create positive associations for him.

"On/Off Button" or "Start Button"

Clicker trainers think of this kind of exercise as a way to offer an animal a choice about whether or not to participate in what you're asking him to do. If he chooses to touch you, that's a way for him to say, "Okay, I'm ready, you can start." It's a way for you to confirm that he's willing to go along with what's coming next—and by the same token, breaking contact can be thought of as a way for him to ask for the session to end. So you can think of this as an "on/off button," which the animal can use thanks to the training that taught him how to touch a target.[55] I've framed it as a "stop" button, because in the context of these exercises, it's a way for you to ask the animal to hold still and not do other things. But there are multiple other ways to look at it, and I invite you to explore the work of other professionals and find out more. In all cases, though, a trainer has to pay close attention to the animal's demeanor and bearing, because an animal who has had enough may simply decide to try to escape the interaction completely. Obviously that reaction is also important information; it means something's gone wrong somewhere in the relationship between animal and trainer, and in the context of training intended to allow you to provide care, it's essential for the animal's health, and even his survival, that he cooperate with assessment and treatment. If you are too focused on the urgency of care, however, you risk demanding too much of your animal, and asking him for more than he can give you. The only guide you really have is his behavior—any sign of fear or avoidance of the procedure needs to be taken seriously.

Touching the Gums

What's the Point?

Touching a horse's gums allows you to check his capillary refill time. Vets will briefly press the tip of one finger to a horse's gums, which will turn pale with the pressure; seeing how long it takes for the normal color to return is useful diagnostic information. A time of several seconds or longer can indicate a problem. This kind of check might be necessary in a case of colic, or to assess a horse's recovery after a major effort (an endurance competition, for example).

What You Want the Horse to Do

- Stay still while a vet spreads his lips apart and presses on his gum.

✦ What You Do

As with most of these exercises, it's best if you're able to do this with the horse free to move, on a loose lead rope, in a familiar place. Start by yourself, and then ask another person to carry out the same set of steps before the big day when the vet is going to come.

You can make this easier with a light restraining hold on the noseband of the horse's halter: place one hand on the bottom of the noseband, with the other moving the lip and contacting the gum (see page 59). The lead should be draped across the horse's neck or in the hand that's holding onto the halter; be careful not to wrap it around your fingers.

✦ Step by Step: Clicker Training and Approach-Retreat

You can follow the steps described here using an approach-withdrawal method without clicks or rewards. But I like to use rewards for this; this exercise is pretty simple, and it's a good opportunity for you and your horse to practice working with the clicker. Food rewards also help your horse form positive associations with having his gums touched.

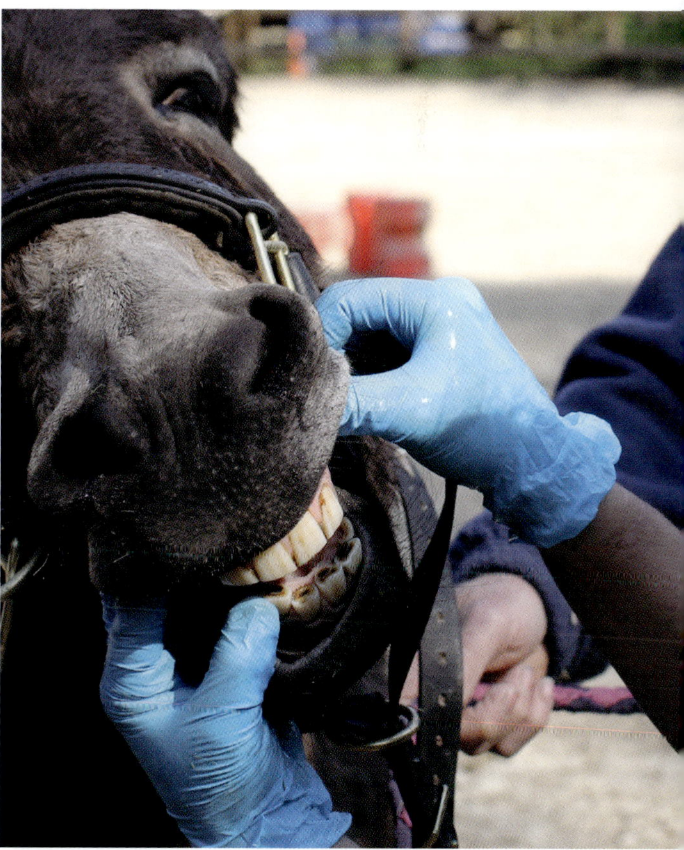

Lifting the horse's lips allows a vet to check the color of his mucus membranes and the condition of his teeth.

1. Touch the side of one of the horse's nostrils. If the horse remains still, click, move your hand away, and reward him with food. If you need to hold the halter more firmly to limit his movements, wait, and as soon as he's standing still, release the pressure and click at the same time, and then reward him.

2. Lift his upper lip to the side (at the back of his incisors). If the horse remains still, click, move your hand away, and reward him with food. If you need to hold the halter more firmly to limit his movements, wait, and as soon as he's standing still, release the pressure and click at the same time, and then reward him.

3. Touch the horse's gum for a fraction of a second. Follow the same steps as above if the horse stays still, and if he doesn't.

4. Press on the horse's gum briefly, and follow the same steps as above if the horse stays still, and if he doesn't.

5. Touch the gum longer, pressing for two seconds. Follow the same steps as above if the horse stays still, and if he doesn't.

To prepare your horse even more thoroughly, you can follow the same steps but position yourself almost directly in front of him.

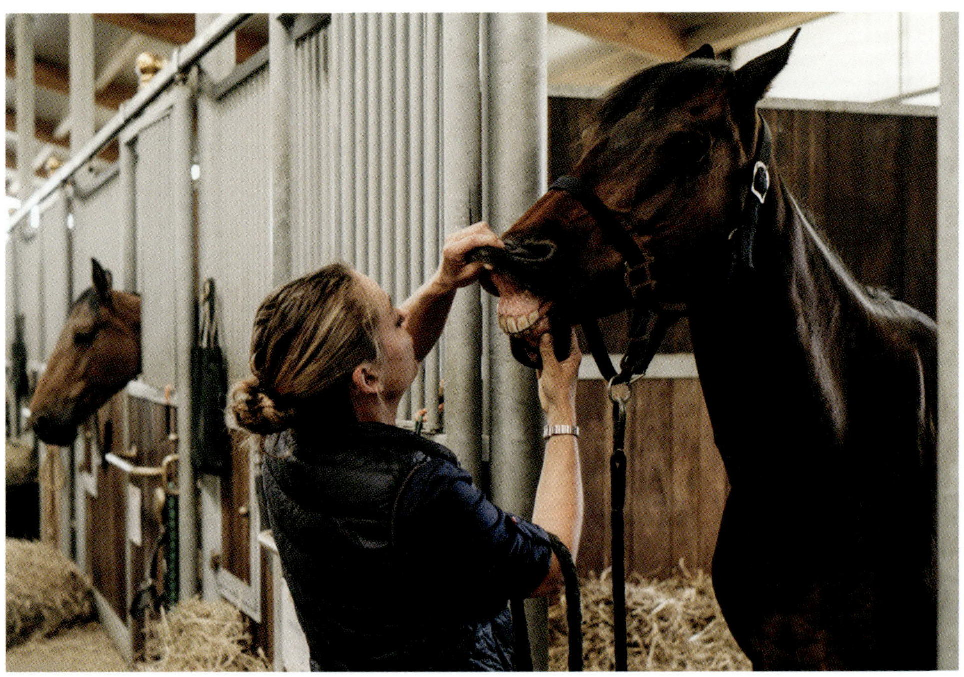

In addition to training on both sides, you can also train the horse from the front. Just look out for your own safety (an upward jerk of the horse's head can catch you in the face if you aren't paying attention).

Watch out for upward jerks of the horse's head toward your face. Shifting your grip to the upper side of the noseband can help you follow any avoidance movements the horse makes, and keep you from getting hit.

The next step is to carry out the same training with a new person, and, as with all of these exercises, to go through these steps in a familiar place and then in an unusual or even wholly new place.

Common Mistakes

- Lifting both of the horse's lips from the front and gripping them (if you've trained your horse to cooperate with a grip on his upper lip, in preparation for potential emergency use of a twitch, he'll have an easier time forgiving this mistake).
- Allowing the contact to break when the horse moves.

◆ Step by Step: The Clicker and Voluntary Contact

You can train the horse to rest his nose—and his upper lip—against the palm of your hand while another person lifts the side of his lip and touches his gum.

When you're working on this, have your helper proceed through stages as for the combination of clicker training and approach-retreat. She needs to stop moving and lift her hand away whenever you click.

To review the approach-retreat technique for touching specific places, refer to Touching Sensitive Places (see page 74). This will allow you to work with horses even if they're very fearful of humans.

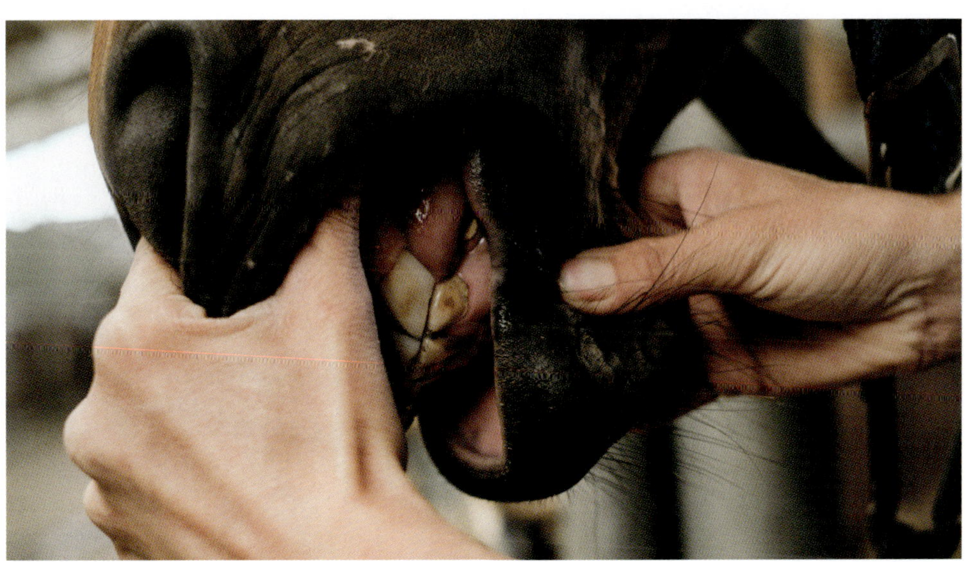

Press on the horse's gum for a few seconds with your thumb.

Taking the Temperature

What's the Point?

Being able to insert a thermometer into a horse's anus with his cooperation allows you to take his rectal temperature. This is more accurate than other methods for measuring body temperature, which is a vital statistic that a vet may need to be able to monitor—for example:

- Before giving the horse a vaccination, to ensure there is no pre-existing infection.

- If the horse is presenting with lameness, in which case an unusually high temperature could be a sign of infection caused by a foreign body in the foot (a nail, for example).

- If the horse is showing dejection and a loss of appetite, which, in conjunction with fever, are early signs of several diseases (piroplasmosis, strangles, rhinopneumonia, and more).

- In cases of unusual weakness, which, with a low temperature, may be hypothermia—in which case, you immediately know you need to cover the horse up and give him a rub to warm him.

It's in your best interest to know how to take your horse's temperature, too, whenever you have doubts about his health. The temperature of an adult horse or donkey at rest should be about 99°–100°F (37°–37.8°C). If your vet isn't able to come out right away, you can still give a clear idea of the potential seriousness of the situation if you know your horse's temperature.

What You Want the Horse to Do

Stay still while his temperature is being taken.

✦ What You Do

You'll do exactly the same thing you did when you were working on Touching Sensitive Places. Three methods are available to you:

- Approach-retreat;

- Clicker and approach-retreat;

- Clicker and target ("stop button").

It's essential that you make sure you can safely touch your horse's hindquarters (rump, haunches, buttocks) before you work on taking his temperature.

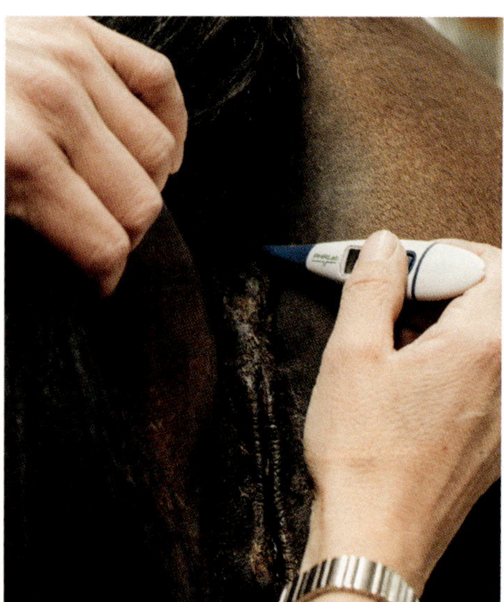

Hold the tail to one side, and hold the thermometer in the other hand.

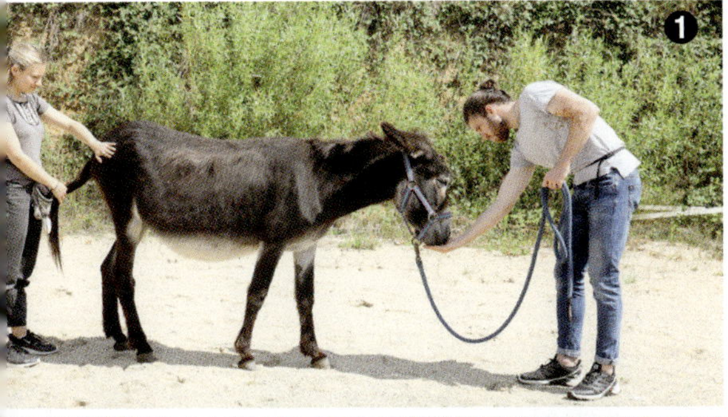

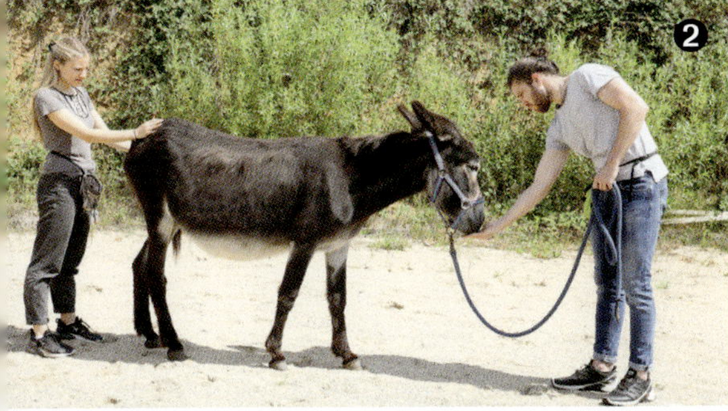

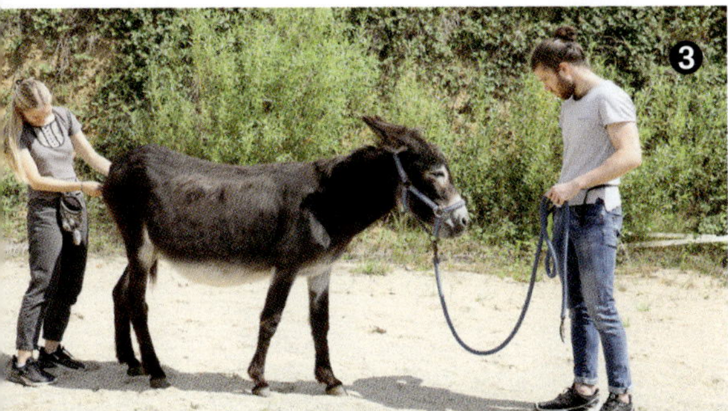

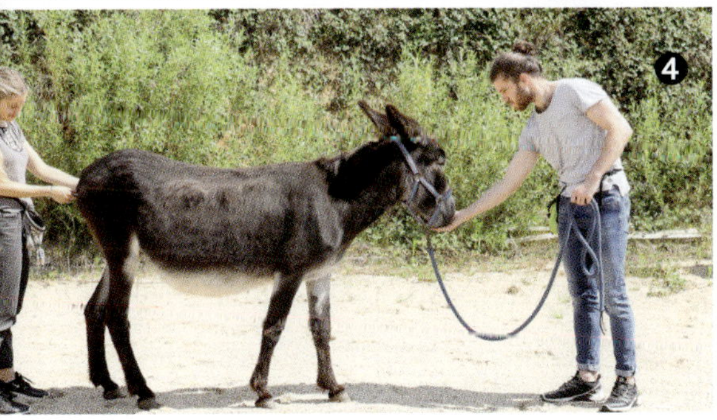

This donkey is trained in stages, and she is rewarded at each stage. A position off to the side instead of directly behind would be safer for the caregiver if she were dealing with a horse; donkeys kick out to the side more readily than they kick straight back, however, so that position directly behind is not especially risky here.

✦ Step by Step

Position yourself to the side, not directly behind your horse. While holding the lead rope, check to make sure you can touch the horse's rump and the backs of his buttocks with your hand held flat. The lead rope should be in the hand that is resting against the horse, with the other hand active. You can also do this exercise with someone else holding the lead rope for you.

1. Touch the top of the horse's tail.

2. Pass your hand between his buttocks and his tail (this is potentially a sensitive place, so go slowly and repeat this until he relaxes).

3. Pass your hand under the tail; lift it slightly if necessary, and touch the area around the anus.

4. Touch the anus itself with the end of the thermometer (if you don't have a rectal thermometer to hand, use another object—the tip of a pen or a plastic syringe will work—so it will feel different from the touch of your hand).

5. Insert the thermometer into the rectum (you may want to lubricate it with petroleum jelly first, as that will make this step easier) for a fraction of a second.

6. Then insert it for a full second.

7. Then keep it there longer and longer, until you can wait all the way until the beep indicating it has taken a reading. Always hold the thermometer firmly with at least two fingers, so the horse

doesn't injure himself if he drops his tail suddenly.

When you've been able to repeat this procedure multiple times and kept the thermometer in place long enough for it to beep each time, you may notice that, if you've been using a clicker and rewards, your horse will raise his tail at the sound of the thermometer beeping, and he'll be waiting for his reward to arrive!

Common Mistakes

• Removing the thermometer whenever the horse moves. For your safety, though, this might be wise! To avoid teaching the horse that movement will get rid of the thermometer for him, break down all the steps as much as possible, and use the combination of the clicker and approach-retreat. Food rewards will go a long way in convincing the horse it's worth it to stand still for this.

✦ Have a Signal for Encouragement

Taking the horse's temperature is a type of contact that has to be sustained, but we can't reward the horse for sustaining it if we're training him alone—no one is going to have an easy time offering a treat to the horse's mouth while holding a rectal thermometer in position at the same time. What you need here is a *secondary reinforcer* (this is the technical term for it in the field of learning theory), which will let you tell the horse he's doing the right thing and that he has to keep

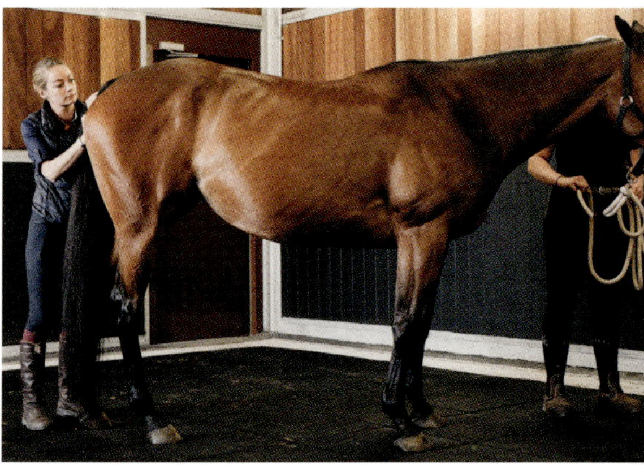

Doing this exercise with two people makes everything simpler.

doing it, until you are able to follow up with the food reward—the *primary reinforcer*. The secondary reinforcer can be a word like, "Yes!" or a touch.

These signals of encouragement can be taught. While studies have shown that horses are sensitive to "baby talk"[56] (also called "pet-directed speech") such as saying, "Yes," or "Bravo," in a high pitch, even if they haven't been trained to understand what it means, it's worth your time to pick a single signal of encouragement and explicitly teach it to your horse, so he'll respond to hearing it even in the middle of a vet's examination. Decide on one or two words, different from whatever marker you're using before you give a food reward (if you chose to use a word or sound instead of a clicker).

Start with an exercise that's already familiar to your horse. Ask him, for example, to touch his nose to a target.

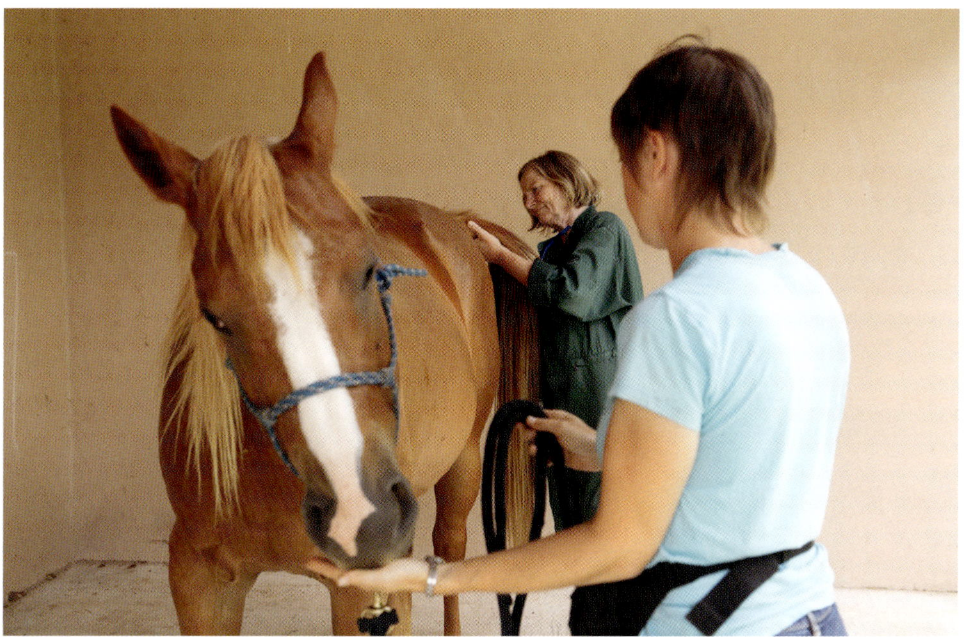

With two people, it's much easier to reward the horse during a temperature measurement, not just after it, as we are doing here with this young horse.

- When he does this exercise correctly—touching the target, in our example here—instead of clicking and rewarding him immediately, use your signal of encouragement ("Yes!"), and then click and reward. Repeat this two or three times, and you should see a very rapid association form, with your horse expecting a reward after the "Yes!" just as much as after the click.

- Then ask again, and when he responds to this request, use the signal of encouragement by itself, but don't follow up with a click, and don't give him a food reward.

- The next time you ask and the horse responds to your request, click and reward.

- Then ask for something from a different, equally familiar exercise—say, doing the Statue, from page 38—and give him the signal of encouragement, followed by a click and a food reward.

Keep alternating like this, without consistently giving a food reward after your signal of encouragement (while still giving it consistently after the click or other marker). Sometimes the signal of encouragement will come with a food reward, and sometimes it won't; this random reinforcement is exactly what makes it powerful.[57] This signal should only be used with behaviors the horse can perform consistently in response to a request, not in the early stages of learning a new behavior.

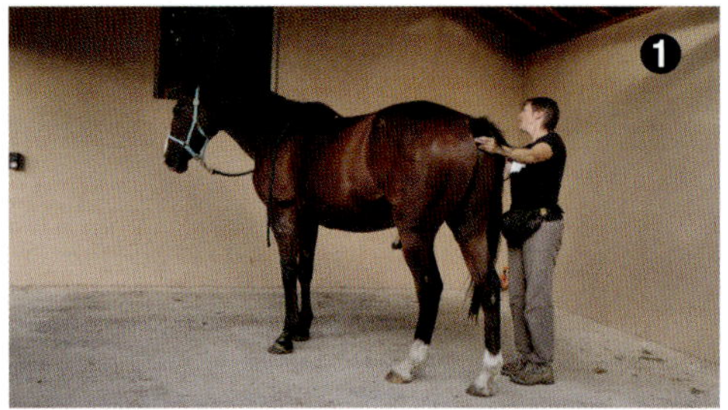
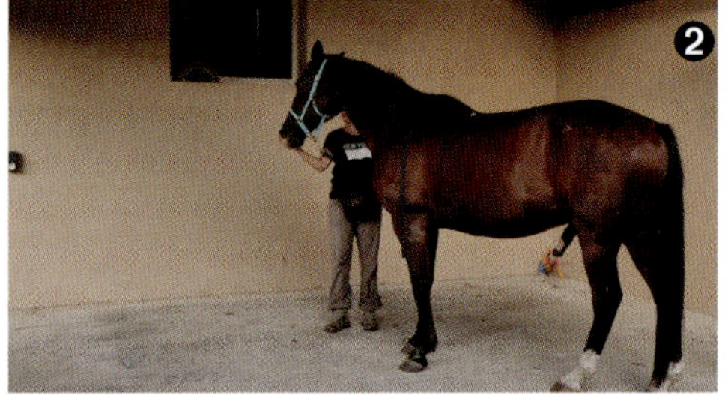

If you're working on this exercise by yourself, you need to have a way to praise your horse for staying still ❶ until you can reward him with food at the end ❷.

Learning from Experience

I had been training a particularly fearful pony for six months with a clicker when, during a veterinary examination, I suddenly realized no one had ever taken his temperature (or at least he'd been very tightly restrained when they had). He jumped at the moment the thermometer was inserted. The vet agreed to wait for a few minutes, and I started from the top, with the step of reaching under the pony's tail. I followed each of the steps described in this exercise, clicking, lifting my hand away, and returning to the pony's head to give him a reward, and the vet didn't have to wait very long before his temperature could successfully be taken. A month later, in advance of a vaccine booster for him, I reviewed this work with him using four rewards and a pipette, because I didn't have a thermometer. When the vet came the next day, the pony didn't move an inch when his temperature was taken; he got a reward during, and then again at the end. (When I work with an animal by myself, I only give a reward at the end, and I use my signals of encouragement to ask for stillness during.)

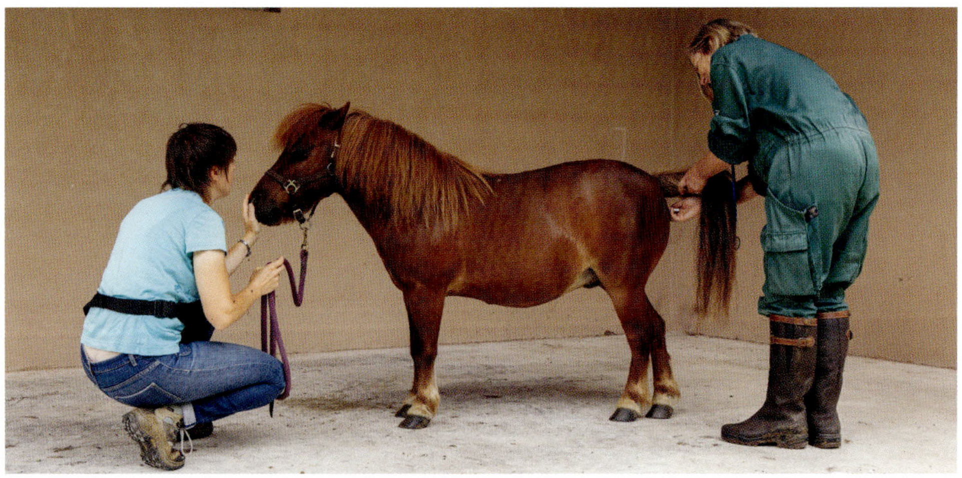

This pony was about to flee, the first time someone tried to take his temperature. With a few minutes of clicker work, though, it was possible to take his temperature with his cooperation.

Clipping

What's the Point?

Clipping isn't just about trimming away a thick coat to keep him cool. Clipping specific areas of the body can be necessary to give access to it for multiple reasons:

- Wound care (cleaning, suturing);
- An ultrasound;
- A blood test, intravenous injection, or catheter insertion;
- Removal of excess coat from a horse or pony with Cushing's syndrome when temperatures are high.

What You Want the Horse to Do

- Stand still when he hears the sound of the clipper running.
- Remain still when the clipper is touching him, while it's running (causing noise and vibrations, along with the sensation of hair falling).

What You'll Need

- A clipper, or a substitute object that can make similar sounds (an electric toothbrush, or at minimum a recording of the sound of a clipper running).

◆ What You Do: Familiarizing Horses with Noise

Getting horses used to the sound of a clipper while it's running is the first step toward being able to clip them, but it doesn't guarantee success. Still, it can make it easier. Consider the following: a researcher set up an experiment in which ponies ate their meals while listening to a recording of a clipper.[58] Six ponies listened to this recording for 10 minutes a day, over 14 days. The sound started right after their food was given to them, and stopped before they were done eating. After those 14 days, these six ponies moved their heads significantly less when they were clipped from the neck upward to the ears.

The advantage of the researcher's technique is that you don't have to actively handle the horses or ponies—you can keep a safe distance. Plus, several animals can be familiarized with the noise at the same time.

Furthermore, with a sound recording, you can control the volume—you can start out with it low, if some horses are too agitated by the normal volume to eat, and then gradually increase it. You just have to be careful to shut off the sound before the horses are done eating.

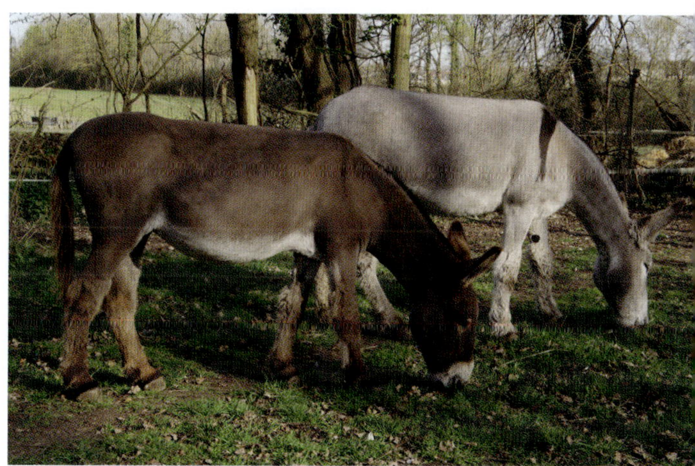

Clipping is sometimes necessary in order to treat skin conditions, like the lice these donkeys had.

So you do still have to be paying attention, in order to observe each animal while the sound is playing, adjust the volume correctly, and stop the recording at the right time.

To train just a few horses who are in neighboring stalls, or one horse alone, you can use an electric toothbrush, which makes a noise a lot like a clipper, and turn it on near the stalls.

Common Mistakes

- Shutting off the sound at the wrong time (if the horse is nervous and stops eating, for example). That will only teach the horse to stop eating in order to make the sound go away, which isn't going to help him get used to the sound.

◆ What You Do: Teaching the Horse to Stand Still While Being Clipped

Several options are available to you depending on how comfortable you are interpreting your horse's expressions and signs of fear or relaxation (see pages 22 to 24 for observable criteria).

If you have trouble spotting different emotions in your horse, or you're worried he'll have a strong reaction (in the form of either escape or aggression), you can work with a helper who can hold him for you. She should stand at his head, slightly to one side (the same side you're standing on). If the horse moves, she can use the lead rope to guide his nose toward both of you at the same time,

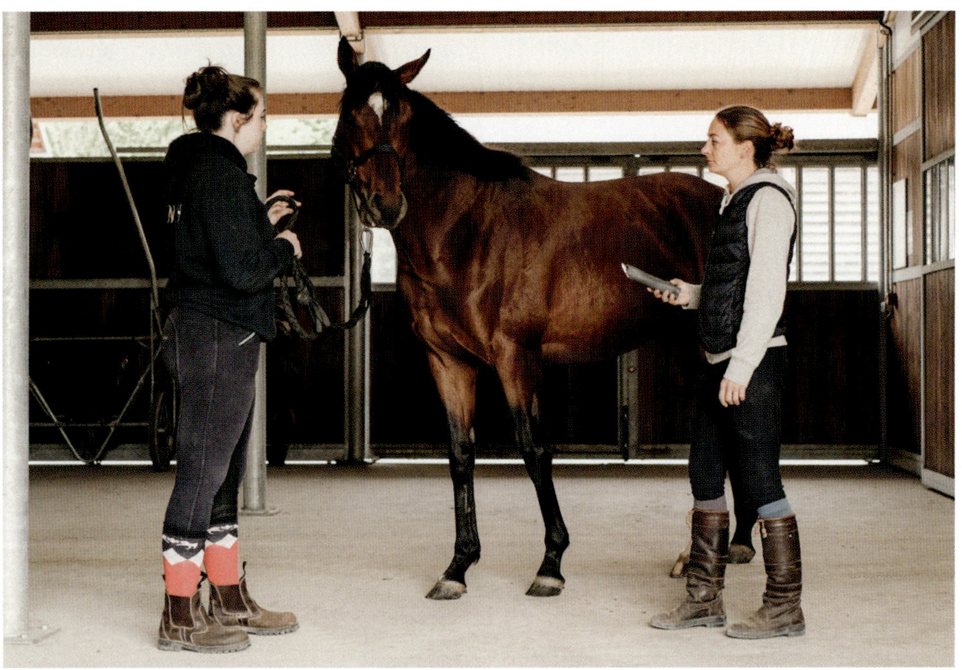

Your helper should hold the lead slack, so it makes a U shape, as long as the horse is standing still. That doesn't mean the lead rope can't be kept relatively short, as it is here.

which will aim his hindquarters away from you and prevent either of you from being kicked. Your helper should keep the lead rope short but slack, allowing it to form a small U as long as the horse is standing still, with his head turned slightly toward the side you're on.

If you're good at handling a long lead rope (12 feet / 4 meters or more) because you do a lot of groundwork, then you can practice this exercise by yourself, with the horse in a halter with a longer lead rope. Start with the clipper, or the sound of one, far enough away from the horse that he accepts it, and be careful to always keep the horse's nose toward you. If your horse is in an environment where he feels calm and you can clearly identify any signs of fear, you can work on this exercise in a relatively large space, allowing the horse to move away from you, but not too far. You do need an enclosed space; a paddock, longeing arena, or riding arena will work, if the horse is used to paying attention to you and staying at your side without you needing to hold him there.

I like to work on this exercise without tying the horse, because that kind of hard limit on his ability to move will tend to make any bad reaction worse—and when I'm not in control of the position of his head, it's harder for me to avoid a kick if I need to.

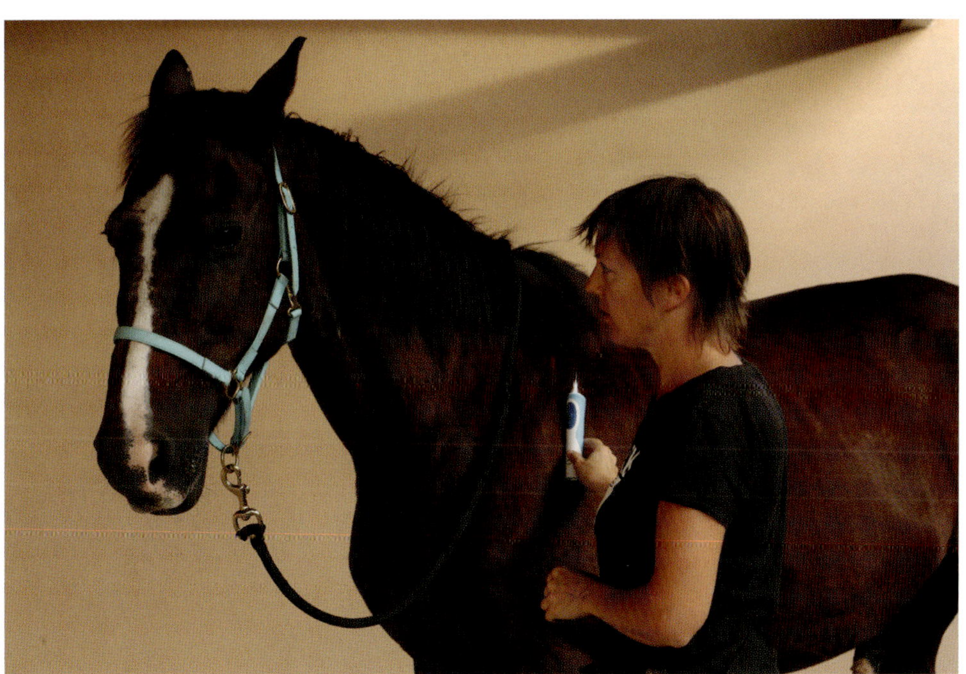

With the lead rope slung over his neck, in a relatively open space, the horse will be less worried about what's happening than he would be if he were confined. You can also keep the lead rope draped over your forearm.

1. Turn on the clipper (or whatever device is available to you to simulate the same kind of noise) far enough away from the horse to allow him to accept it (this could be 30 feet or more, if your horse is nervous about the noise when it's any closer to him than that).

2. Wait for your horse to stand still.

3. Shut off the noise once the horse is standing still, and take a step away.

4. Move closer than before, and repeat.

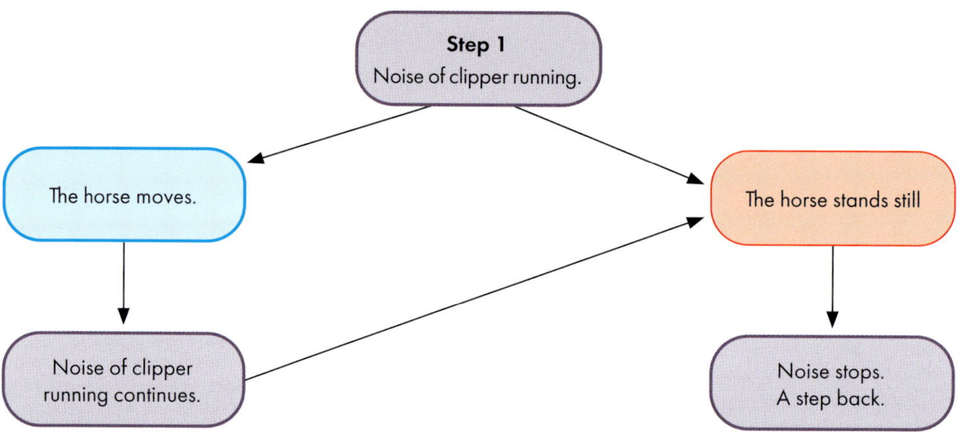

Step 1 in detail.

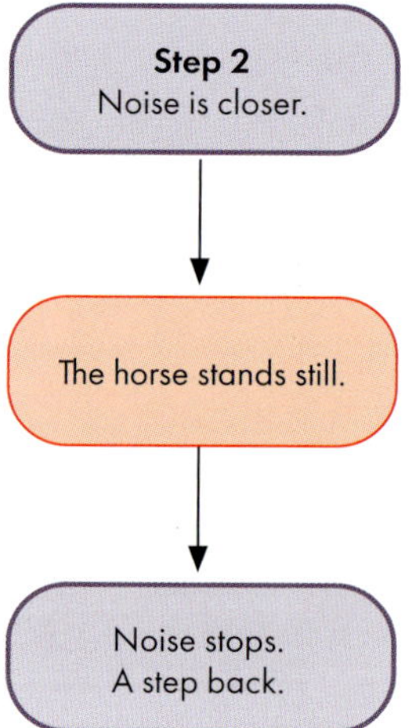

Step 2 in detail.

For each of these steps, you need to stop the noise when your horse is standing still, and then take a step away. This is the "approach-retreat" technique again (see Touching Sensitive Places, page 74). To make it more efficient and more effective, you can combine it with clicker training (see the Statue exercise on page 38 to get started). To do this, when you shut off the clipper or the noise of the clipper and take a step back, you'll also mark the horse's stillness by clicking (with your tongue or by using a word, since you'll have the clipper in one hand and the lead rope in the other, unless you have a helper and a hand free for the clicker). Either your helper who is holding the horse will need to give the food reward, or you'll do it yourself, making sure your horse isn't afraid of the clipper in your hand when it's turned off. If he *is* afraid of it, then set it down before you approach him, give the reward, and then back up and retrieve it.

Don't be greedy; be willing to start as far away from the horse as he needs you to be before you start up the sound of the clipper, toothbrush, or recording. It's better to start a good 45 feet away than to try to start too close and cause a major fear response in your horse. You'll be able to make quicker progress if you respect your horse's degree of tolerance for the noise than if you try to push past it. If you do get too close, start over again from even farther away.

You don't have to complete all the steps in the first session, either.

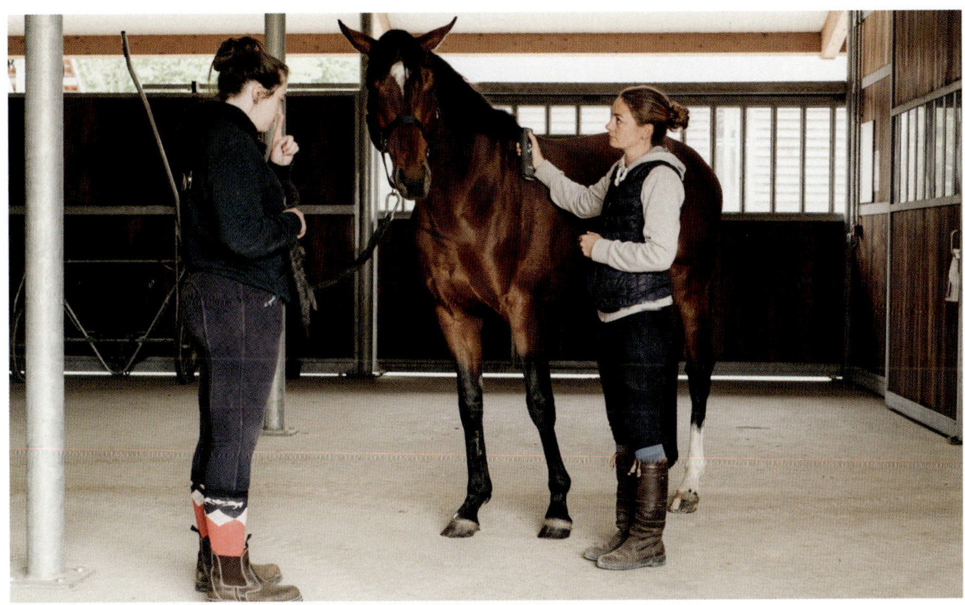

Watch your horse closely to spot signs of fear. Here, this horse's ears are facing downward and extended sideways; he's suspicious, and thinking about moving forward.

It's possible to do it, but pay attention to the limits of both your own patience and the effort your horse is having to put in. Watch him for signs of annoyance (see page 25). If you see any, it's time to take a break. Opt for a short (5 minutes) but quality session—where the horse is able to let you come closer without any fear reactions surfacing—over a long session where you're pushing as far as you can in one day, not least because you risk skipping steps your horse needs.

If you notice more and more reactions from your horse—moving forward, backing up, shaking his head, threatening to bite or kick, flicking his tail, scratching—try backing up to previous steps or reducing the volume of the noise. If that doesn't help, stop the session. If you have to end the session without achieving anything you think is satisfactory, that's too bad. Safety comes first. Think through the reasons why you didn't get the progress you wanted, and come back another day if you've figured out where you went wrong. Otherwise, ask for help.

When the horse is used to the noise, switch to these steps, first with the clipper off and then with it on:

1. Get closer, little by little (one step at a time).

2. Touch the horse with the hand that isn't holding the clipper, and stay still.

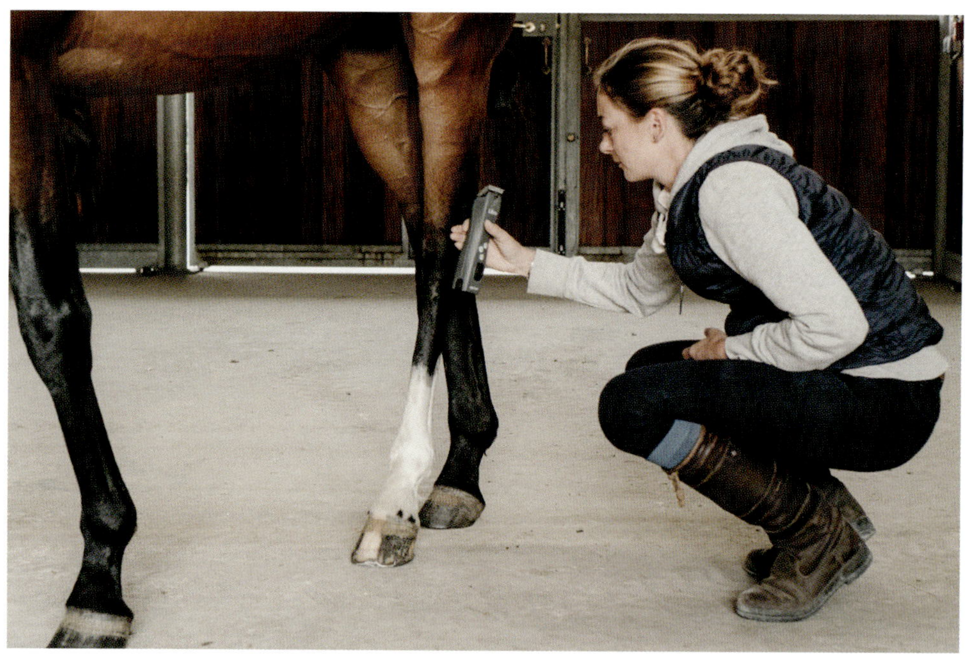

Keeping the flat of your hand between the clipper and the horse's body will reduce the vibrations. For the sake of your safety, though, it would be better to have both hands on the horse's limb, so you can follow his movement if he shifts suddenly and keep yourself clear of it.

 —— PREPARING YOUR HORSE OR DONKEY FOR VETERINARY CARE

3. Touch the neck, and hold the clipper against the shoulder.

4. Keep the clipper in the same spot for a longer duration.

5. Make large, slow movements toward another area.

6. Move from the neck down the back, to the top of the rump.

7. Move from the neck down toward the hip.

8. Move toward the head and then back to a neutral area.

You should only consider actually clipping your horse after at least three sessions like this, with the clipping on the fourth.[59] You'll be able to make sure the training has sunk in, and you should observe more relaxation from your horse over the course of those three sessions (blinking, lowering the head, relaxing the tail).

Learning from Experience

UK equine training professional Gemma Pearson has reached every milestone of this clipping exercise with a pony who used to rear whenever he was clipped, over the course of 24 approach-retreat sessions without using food rewards. It took 6 minutes, with the pony in a halter being held by a second person; the pony initially showed avoidance reactions.

You can see the demonstration video, part of the "Don't Break Your Vet!" series, titled "Calm Clipping," by scanning the QR code to the right.

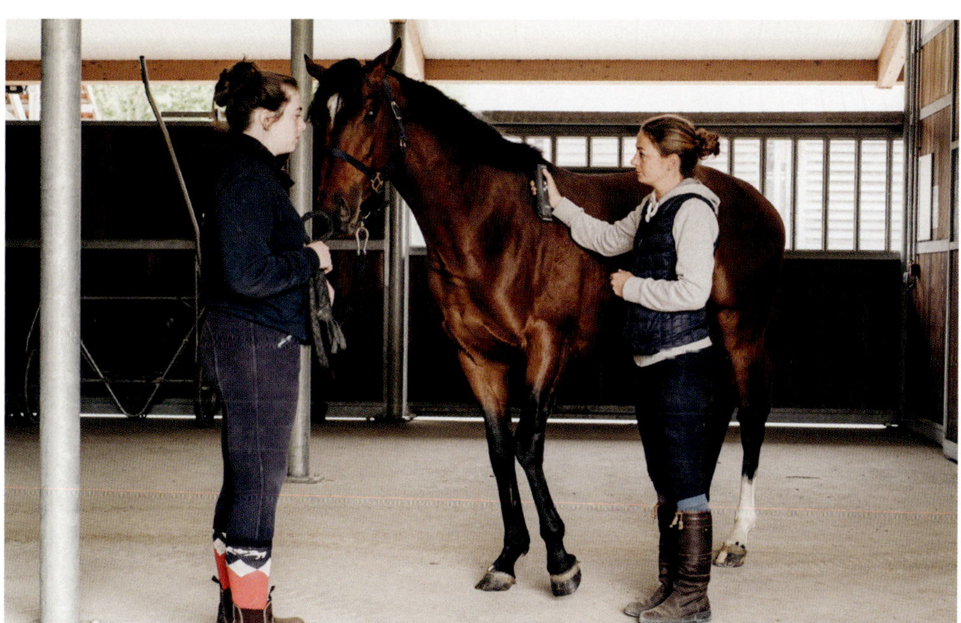

The mistake here would be to break off the contact of the clipper while the horse is moving. On the contrary—you should only break contact when the horse is standing still, so he learns moving won't make the clipper go away.

Common Mistakes

- Shutting off the noise of the clipper when the horse moves
- Leaving the noise at the same intensity while the horse is showing strong fear reactions.

✦ Step by Step: The Clicker and Approach-Retreat

You can follow the same steps as for approach-retreat in general, and add in the clicker: click when the horse stands still, and then move away and return to him with a food reward. Refer to Touching Sensitive Places for more details on combining these techniques (see page 74).

During the clipping process, if you're holding the horse and someone else is doing the clipping, you can reward him easily while he's standing still. If you're clipping by yourself, then it's a good idea to teach your horse a signal of encouragement you can use to tell him he's doing the right thing and you appreciate his patience, but you can't reward him for it right away. See page 90 for details on signals of encouragement, and take breaks to give him rewards several times during the clipping.

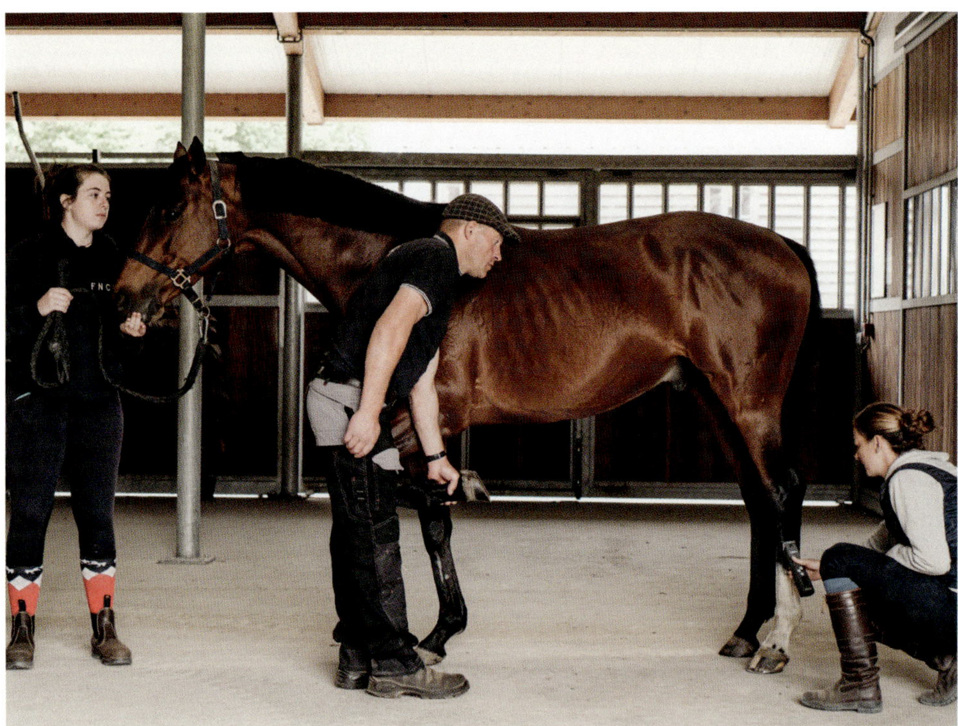

When you're clipping sensitive areas like the limbs, you can restrain the horse with a foreleg hold on the same side, to help keep him absolutely still—and you can reward him at the same time. It's a good idea for the person doing the clipping to have both hands in contact with the horse, one still and steady and the other handling the clipper, in order to keep the movements of the clipper smooth and avoid startling the horse.

This approach is good for especially sensitive horses. It requires more of an upfront time investment, but it makes it much easier for you to check in with your horse and make sure you haven't exceeded the requests he can handle. You'll need two people for this approach. Refer to Touching Sensitive Places for more information about how to proceed (see page 74).

Your horse should have learned, over the course of around four sessions, to touch his nose to your palm, keep it there, and stand still, even with another person touching him or palpating parts of his body. During a fifth session, introduce a new element: have your helper touch the horse with the clipper while it's turned off. If this step is too difficult for your horse because he has strong negative associations with the clipper, go back to contact without the clipper involved, with a free hand and then with a neutral object (a brush, for example). Then try again, introducing the clipper more gradually—for example, instead of proceeding with only two or three attempts in between presenting the clipper to the horse and touching him with it, do it in 10 micro-steps. Do the same, preferably across multiple sessions, with the clipper turned on.

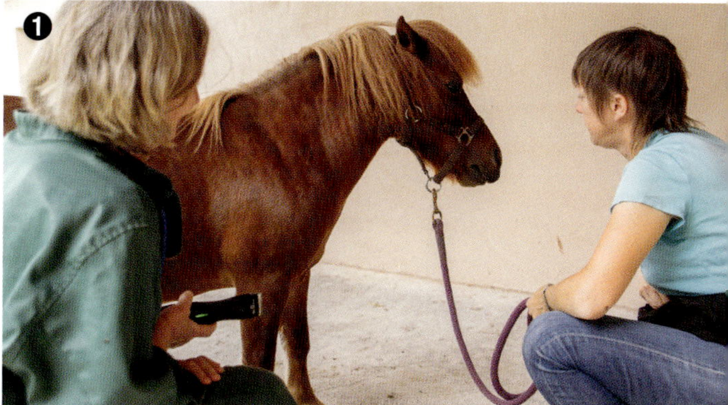

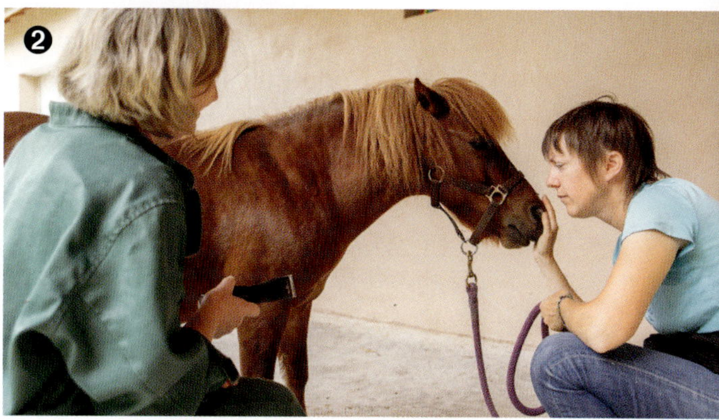

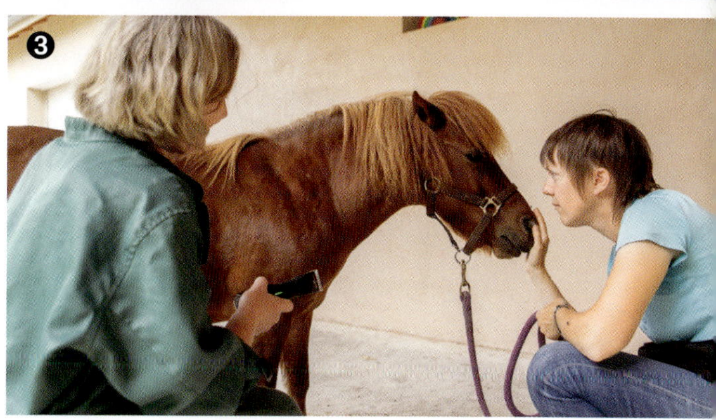

❶ The pony, already familiar with the noise of the clipper, shows a fear reaction here that's actually about the presence of the veterinarian (raising his head and neck).

❷ We shut off the clipper and see whether he holds still the veterinarian present with the clipper off. He does, and I click my tongue and reward him.

❸ The pony keeps his contact with my hand, so the veterinarian turns the clipper back on for 2 seconds and then turns it off again. This is short enough that the pony doesn't feel the need to break contact, and I click and reward him again.

Bathtime

What's the Point?

Being able to bathe a horse with his cooperation lets you do things like clean wounds, promote circulation in swollen limbs, and remove clay poultices. It's also helpful to allow a veterinarian to properly examine the limbs of a lame horse—and your farrier will appreciate it, too. It's not easy to feel or see an injury on a muddy leg. Plan to do this a little in advance of the vet's visit, so the horse's limbs aren't overly cool from the evaporating water; abnormal temperatures, whether high or low, are potential diagnostic criteria. For an ordinary vet check, washing the horse's legs at the minimum is essential.

After surgical castration or when the horse has a wound, pain or sensitivity in the relevant area might cause the horse to want to avoid water; the genital area is often extra sensitive in general, too, even when nothing is wrong. Horses can also get nervous about the jet of water moving around them, the shape of the hose coiling on the ground, and contact with the water itself.

What You Want the Horse to Do

- Stand still with all four feet on the ground while he's being bathed.

✦ What You Do

When it comes to the location for this exercise, you won't have as much choice as usual, since you need a

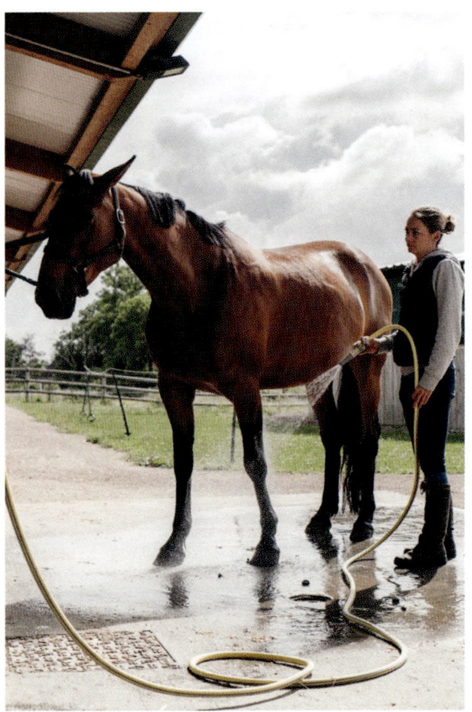

Be aware that a coiling ground hose might frighten your horse in and of itself, whether there's water spraying out of it or not. Train him to accept it by gradually moving it closer to him.

hose with a water supply. You can work alone, holding the lead rope yourself, or ask someone to help you. As with the clipping exercise, make sure you and your helper are both on the same side of the horse, and bring his nose toward both of you to avoid a kick. For safety's sake, it's better to work with a horse who is free to move; the more confined the horse feels in the face of a possible threat, the more violently he'll tend to react to it.

✦ Step by Step

Follow the same fundamental steps as for Clipping. Three techniques are available to you:

- Approach-retreat;
- Clicker and approach-retreat;
- Clicker and target ("stop button").

I'll run through the steps briefly here; for more details on the principles you need to apply for each of the three techniques, refer to the Clipping exercise (see page 93). At each stage, stop what you're doing as soon as the horse stands still, and move the jet of water away from him. If you choose a technique involving food rewards, when the horse stands still, click (or mark the behavior using whatever marker you've chosen), move the jet of water away, and reward the horse with the food. It'll be easier to practice this exercise with a helper, because sometimes when you let go of a hose, it will move around unpredictably thanks to the water pressure, which can frighten even a horse who didn't mind the hose while you were holding it. If your water pressure is relatively low, though, you won't have this problem, and you can work alone.

1. Reward the horse for standing still in the area where you're going to bathe him.
2. Turn the water on with the hose at a distance from the horse (3 feet or more), with a low flow.
3. Turn on the water, bring the hose and jet of water a little closer to the horse, and wait for the horse to stand still again; as soon as he does, move the water away from him.
4. Repeat, bringing the hose closer.
5. Wet part of one of the horse's legs, and keep the spray pointed at his leg for as long as he is still moving (starting with a front leg here will be easier than starting with a hind leg); once he is standing still, move it away.
6. Start wetting the leg again for a second at a time.
7. Increase the duration of the spray against the leg.
8. Start moving the spray up and down the length of the leg.
9. Follow the same steps for a hind leg.
10. Increase the water pressure a little more, and repeat.

Each step must be repeated as many times as it takes for your horse to grow comfortable with it and become willing to stand still. Keep going until the horse has stood still twice in a row

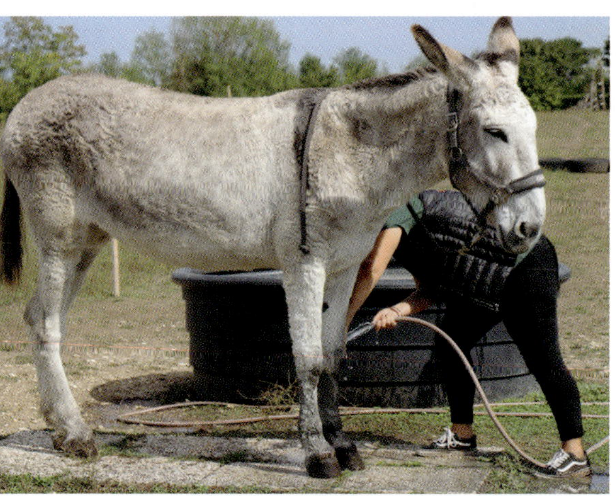

When you're training your equine, start with the front legs rather than the hind legs. Here, this donkey learned to stand still while he was being bathed, and to stay in the designated place, on the slabs.

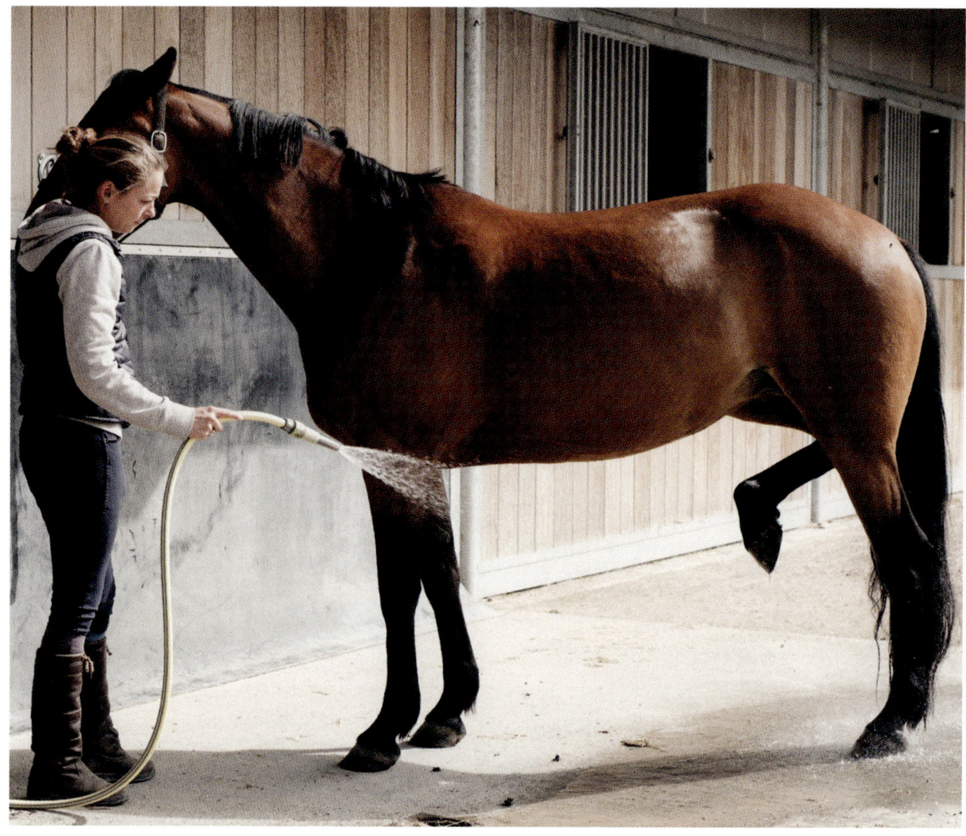

Here, it's important to keep following this mare's rising hind foot with the jet of water, in order to avoid teaching her that dodging the water will make it go away.

at each stage before you move on to the next. These steps can take place over as many sessions as you need.

The movement of a hose on the ground can frighten your horse. If you end up in this situation, you'll also have to work on giving the horse a chance to accept the movement of the hose, both when there isn't water touching him and when there is. Start with small movements of the hose, and then larger ones. Some horses are less afraid of a hose that's wrapped up on a reel, but that's not always an option.

I've discussed washing the legs. To bathe other parts of the body, you'll have to be able to pass the water over it first. If your horse is sensitive or might be sensitive at the moment (because of a wound, for example), practice approach-retreat as described in Touching Sensitive Places, on page 74; imagine the spray of water is your hand, and everything else will be pretty much the same. Including clicks and rewards will make the process more pleasant for the horse.

Common Mistakes

- Breaking off the contact of the water with one of the horse's legs when the horse raises the leg. You need to maintain contact, and not move the water away until the horse has set his leg back down.
- Breaking off the contact of the water when the horse moves around.

Applying a Spray

What's the Point?

Sprays and aerosol products may be used to:

1. Disinfect wounds;
2. Apply fly repellent so the horse isn't shifting around during examination or treatment;
3. Apply a product to the skin (an antifungal treatment, for example);
4. Detangle hair … although that's more a matter of grooming than veterinary care!

What You Want the Horse to Do

- Hold still while a spray is applied.

What You'll Need

- Instead of wasting an actual skincare product or fly spray, find an empty spray bottle you can fill with water—maybe a used-up gardening

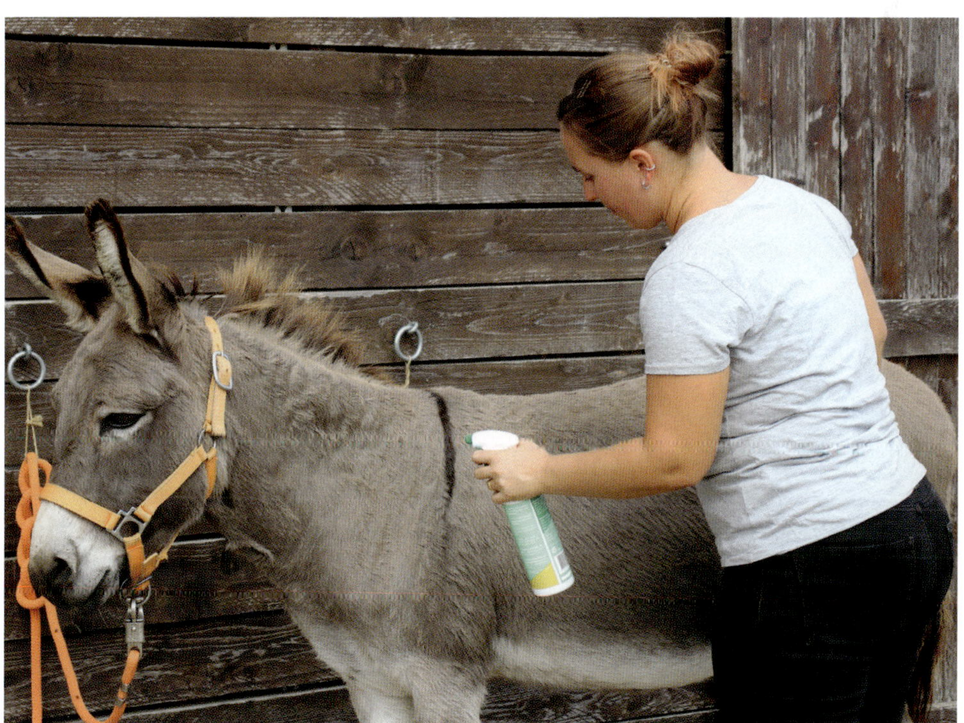

This donkey has learned to stand still while a spray is used, so it's not a problem for his lead rope to be tied the way it is, with a loop of weak twine. However, while you're working on this exercise, it's better to do it with a loose lead rope.

spray, or a leftover bottle from a refillable deodorant or perfume.

✦ What You Do

You can practice this exercise on your own, holding the lead rope yourself, or you can ask someone to help you. If you have a helper, make sure both of you are standing on the same side of the horse, and keep his head angled slightly toward that side to help avoid a kick. For safety's sake, don't tie the horse; the more confined he is in the face of a potential threat, the more violently he might react to it.

Both the noise of the spray being spritzed and the sensation of wet droplets landing on their hair can make horses nervous. And the spray bottle itself, if past experience has led a horse to identify it as an object worth fearing, can also be a problem. All of these possibilities should be addressed in this training.

✦ Step by Step

To familiarize the horse with the noise of the spray bottle, follow the same fundamental steps as for Clipping, with your choice of three techniques:

- Approach-retreat;
- Clicker and approach-retreat;
- Clicker and target ("stop button").

You'll have to squeeze repeatedly on the bottle's trigger for as long as the horse keeps moving. Strengthen your fingers!

To familiarize the horse with the sensation of the spray touching him, I have three tips for you, drawn from the experiences of other trainers who've struggled with this element:

- Aim for the tips of the hair for the first spray toward the horse's body, so the sensation of wetness and contact will be very light.

- Apply the product (or the water, during your training sessions) to your hand first, and then stroke the horse with a flat palm, in the same direction as his hair, along his neck or shoulder. You can also use a sponge and protect your hand with a glove, depending on the product.

- Spray equipment that will cover the horse's body—spray a saddle pad or blanket with fly spray, for example—instead of spraying the horse with the product directly.

You can also teach the horse a word that warns him the spray is coming—"Spray!" or "Look out!" Studies have demonstrated that a consistent warning cue like this before a potentially unpleasant event reduces the degree of surprise and distress animals experience.[60]

I encourage you to click and reward after the first spritz, and then do it again. If your horse stands still for a spritz twice in a row, you can try spraying more of his body. Start with the shoulders, and avoid moving toward the eyes and ears.

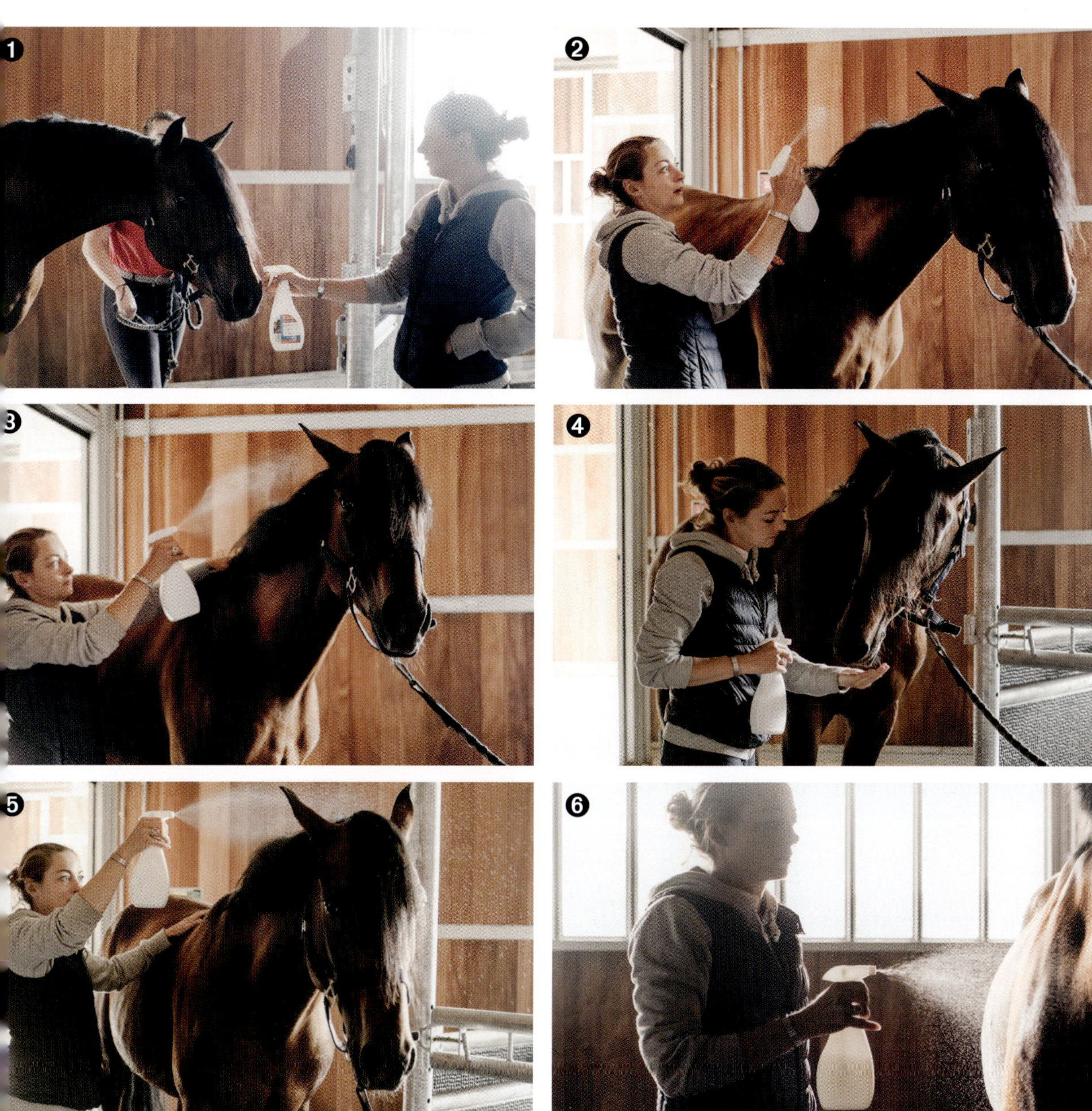

Progressing step by step, using voluntary contact and approach-retreat: Touch the spray bottle without squeezing the trigger; click and reward ❶. The noise of the spray often worries the horse. You can warn him with a word to avoid surprising him with it. Here, you can see that the whites of this horse's eyes are visible and his ears are facing backward—he is afraid ❷. Having the spray directed toward his ears worries this horse even more; his eyes are wider, and he's tensed his neck ❸. Even though he's worried, he doesn't move his feet, and he gets a reward ❹. He's still a little worried, but he's started to relax—the whites of his eyes aren't visible anymore, and he's lowered his head ❺. We end on an easier area—here, the shoulder—and then we'll reward him again ❻.

Preparing for Dental Care

What's the Point?

Dental work for horses is usually done by veterinarians or equine dental technicians. You won't be carrying out these treatments yourself, and you won't be able to prepare the horse for absolutely everything—but that only makes training more important.

In some places, only vets are allowed to sedate an equine to calm him down before dental work is done. This helps minimize the reaction of the horse, pony, or donkey to the treatment. Equine dental technicians, by contrast, aren't typically allowed to administer tranquilizers, and have to work without it. Either way, training your horse to accept the movements and objects used to carry out dental work can help keep him calm and make procedures easier on the big day.

It's worth it to have your horse's mouth and teeth checked every year, or at least every two years, by a professional; horses' teeth grow continuously throughout their lives, unlike human teeth, and uneven patterns of wear can create problem spots or even injuries to a horse's cheeks and tongue. These kinds of issues can have all kinds of impacts:

- Chewing will be harder and won't work as well, which will make the horse's food more difficult for him to digest fully—an especially serious problem for an older horse, because he risks losing more weight than he can afford.
- Any work that involves equipment on the horse's head, whether it's in hand or under saddle, with a bit or without one, may press his cheeks against overgrown or uneven teeth, leading to increasing discomfort and seeming "misbehavior" in response to it.
- An infection in even a single tooth can cause sinusitis, with potentially grave consequences for the horse's overall health.

What You Want the Horse to Do

- Stand still with his mouth open or half-open during dental treatment.
- Learn not to be afraid of or uncomfortable with having his mouth examined.

✦ What You Do

You can practice this exercise on your own, holding the lead rope yourself. For safety's sake, don't tie the horse; the more confined he is in the face of a potential threat, the more violently he might react to it.

Training your horse to stay calm while his mouth is handled or rinsed, while there are vibrations next to him or against his head, and while there are metal objects in his mouth will help prepare him for dental work even if you don't have specialized equipment like a dental rasp to use on him.

If you've already done some of the other exercises to prepare for different kinds of care, you'll know there are multiple approaches you can take to this training. In this case,

I strongly recommend that you use clicker training, which is the clearest way to help your horse understand what's expected of him, and also gives him a straightforward motivation to cooperate (food rewards).

Dental care usually involves fairly lengthy procedures, which makes it difficult to provide food rewards during—and of course food also makes something of a mess in the mouth, right where the dental professional is trying to work. So creating a history of pleasant experiences similar to these treatments is your best bet for keeping your horse in a cooperative frame of mind. Check out the basic exercises in chapter 2 to learn how to start using food rewards correctly. You can also use a signal of encouragement to support your horse, pony, or donkey during a long procedure where you can't directly reward him (see page 90).

What You'll Need

- An electric toothbrush;
- A bit, either the right size for the horse or a larger size;
- A syringe filled with water, without a needle (50 ml, if you have it, since that's the most common size used in dental work, but 30 ml will do in a pinch).

◆ Step by Step: The Clicker and Approach-Retreat

Manipulate the Mouth

Use the Touching the Gums exercise to help your horse accept contact in this area (see page 85). You can add a

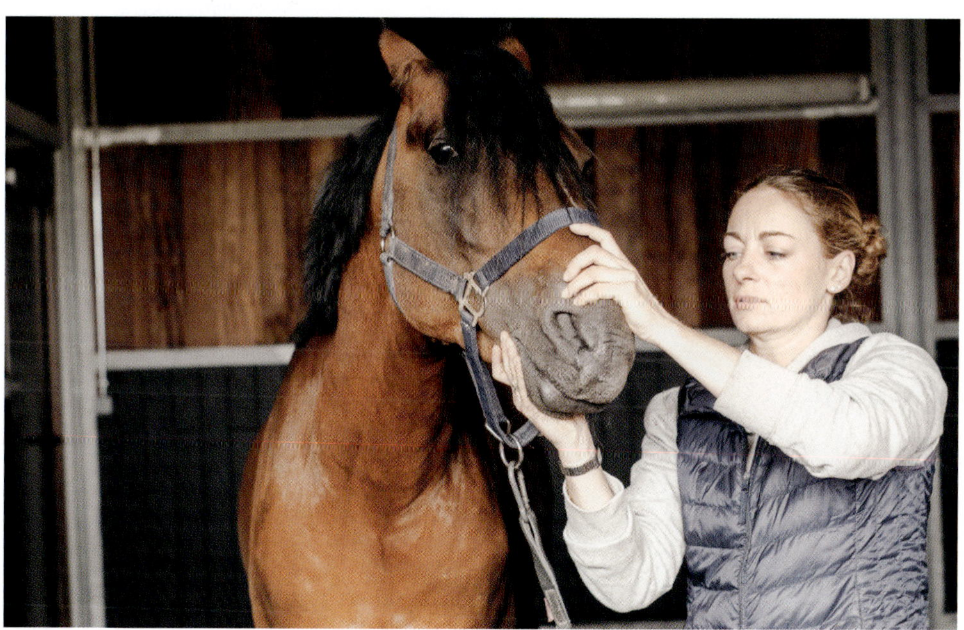

Gently manipulate the lower jaw; click; release; and reward.

step to it for this purpose—keep practicing spreading the lips a little further to the sides than that exercise required.

The exercise Using a Twitch will also be useful here, because equine dental professionals will check dental occlusion by parting the horse's lips from the front (see page 69). You can add two more steps to practice, in this case:

- Grasp the lower jaw, and lift the upper lip;
- Grasp the lower jaw, and move it gently right and left, side to side.
- Teach your horse to accept this kind of contact for a few extra seconds.

Noise and Vibration

To help familiarize a horse with a specific noise, follow the steps for any of the techniques outlined in the Clipping exercise that use an electric toothbrush (see page 93). For this, you only need the handle of an electric toothbrush. When the horse is willing to hold still with the toothbrush running about a foot away from him, add the following steps:

1. Touch his shoulder with your hand closed around the toothbrush.

2. Touch his shoulder with the toothbrush directly.

3. Shift the point of contact for this touch gradually up his neck …

4. … until you're touching the toothbrush to his cheek.

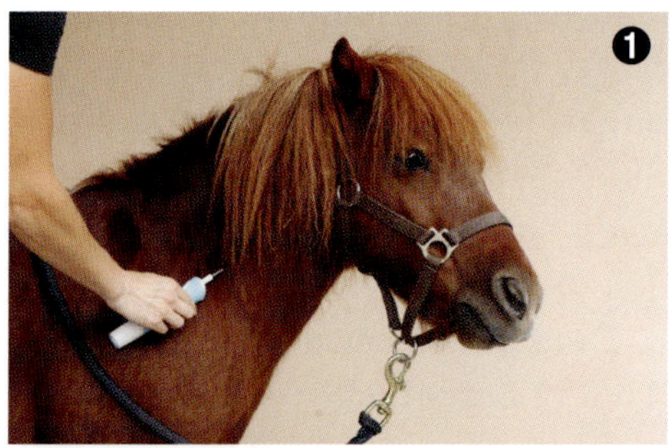
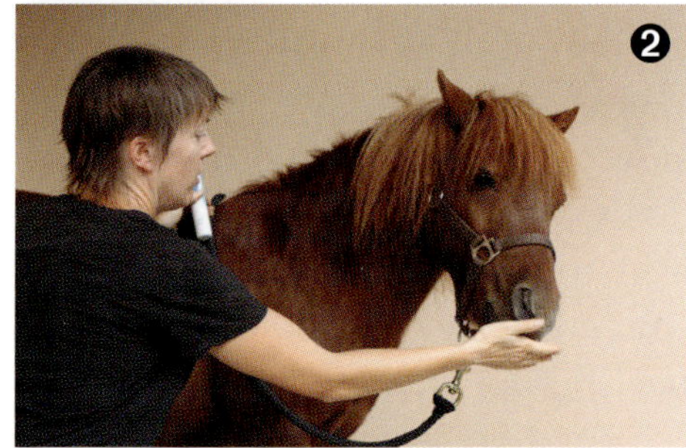

Step 2: Touch the shoulder with the vibrating toothbrush ❶. Reward each step ❷.

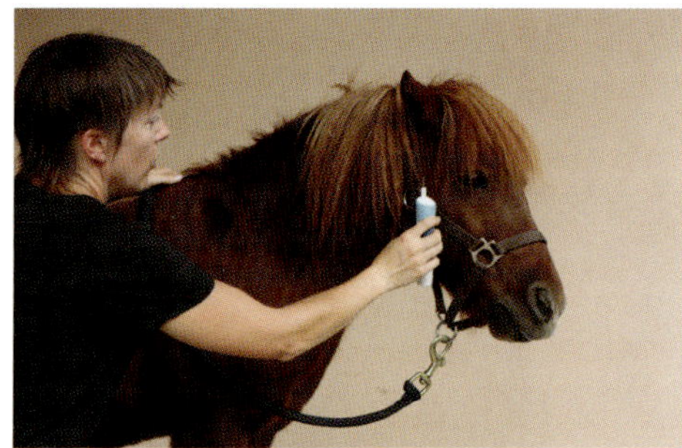

Step 4: Touching the upper cheek with the toothbrush.

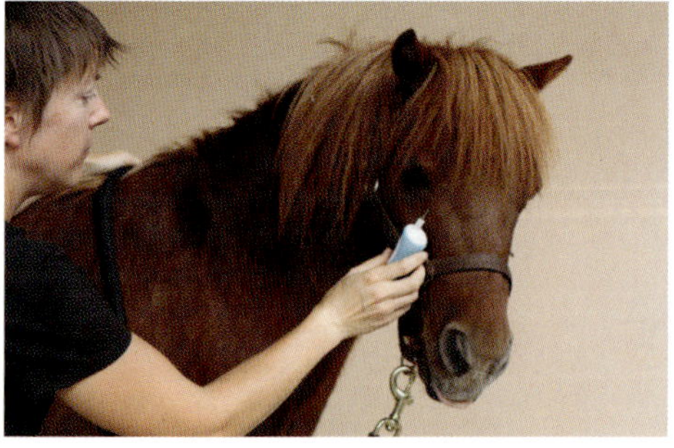

Step 5: Touching various parts of the cheek, until the pony is willingly accepting the touch himself.

 — PREPARING YOUR HORSE OR DONKEY FOR VETERINARY CARE

5. Touch different areas of the cheek until the horse is willing to accept the vibration all over.

It's a good idea to train your horse this way on both sides of his body. If he reacts badly to the vibrations once the toothbrush is touching his head, you can add another step, holding the toothbrush so your hand is between it and the horse's head to dampen the vibrations.

Rinsing the Mouth

Refer to the Administering a Dewormer exercise (see page 130) for more detail on specific steps. The addition here will be using the clicker technique to mark the behavior you want and let the horse know when he's earned a reward. As a final step, use a syringe filled with water, without a needle, and rinse the horse's mouth several times, rewarding him each time if he holds still.

Metal in the Mouth

You can use a metal bit to simulate the kinds of tools equine dental professionals use to hold a horse's mouth open. A horse who's accustomed to a metal bit won't be upset about having an object like this in his mouth, but it's still worth practicing—food rewards, given consistently in response to behavior you're asking for, can only improve your relationship with your horse, which will make any unexpected difficult situations easier for you both to handle. For horses who *aren't* used to a bit, this part of the exercise will help them accept having a chilly piece of metal in their mouths and adjust to the sensation of it against their teeth.

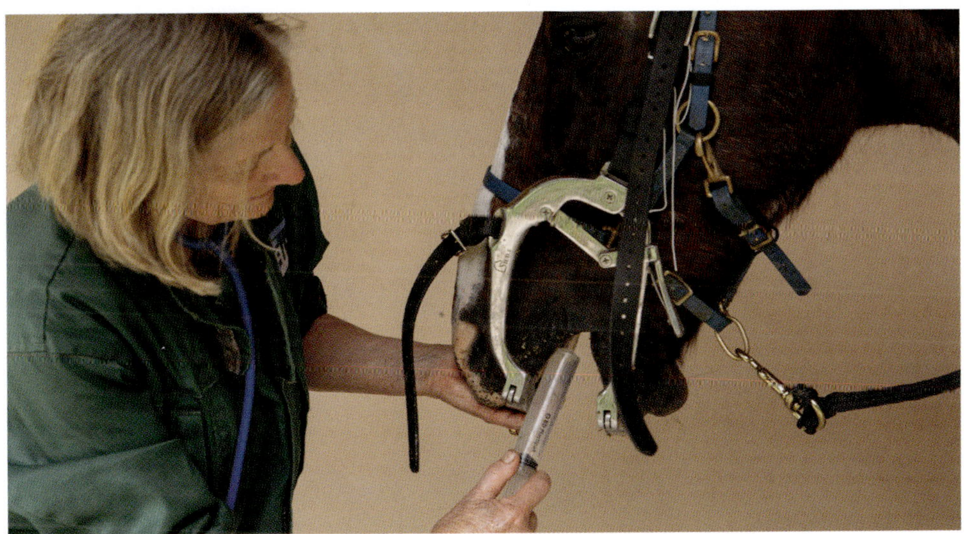

Training your horse to accept having water sprayed into his mouth to rinse it will help him worry less about it on the day he needs dental work.

You can use the approach-retreat technique, or present the bit to the horse as a target for him to touch with his nose (see page 47). The fundamental steps will be the same either way:

1. Touch/ask the horse to touch the bit at the level of his upper lip.

2. Increase the duration of the contact.

3. Insert the bit between the horse's lips without continuing between the teeth.

4. Insert the bit and place it behind the incisors (the space without teeth, right in front of the premolars).

5. Insert the bit and remove it again, letting it strike the incisors lightly on the way.

6. Insert the bit farther, between the premolars.

7. Leave the bit between the premolars for a longer duration.

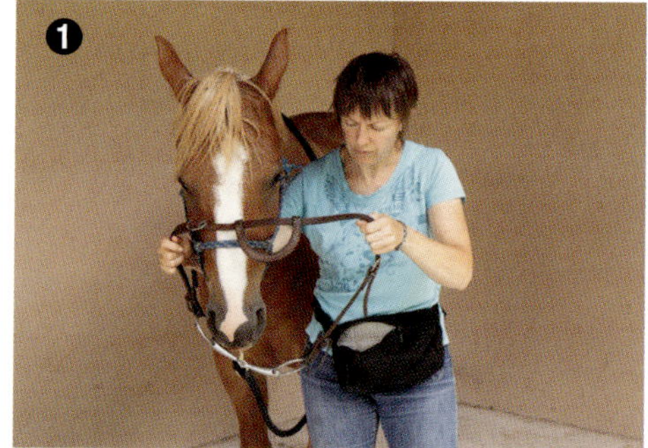

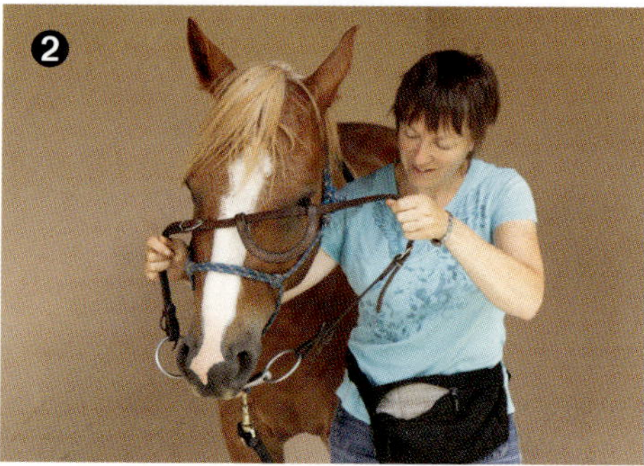

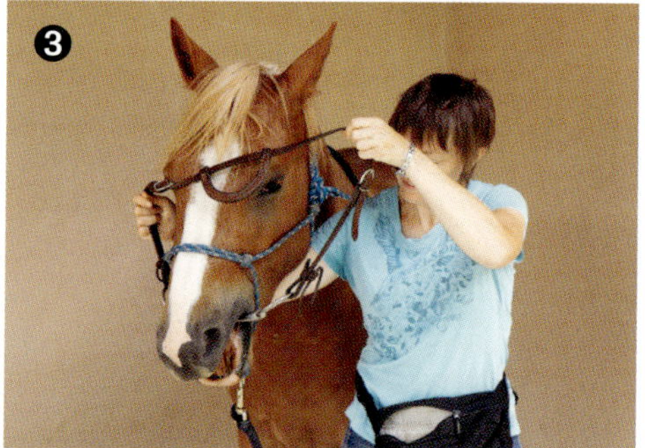

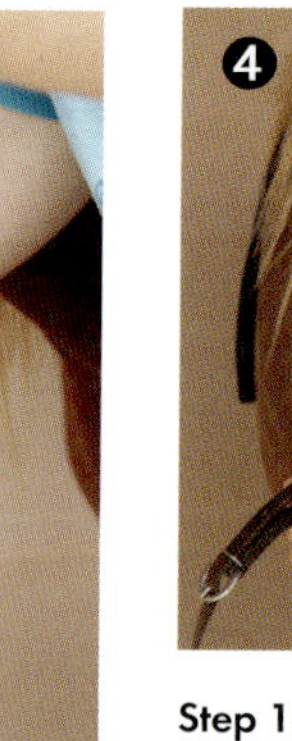

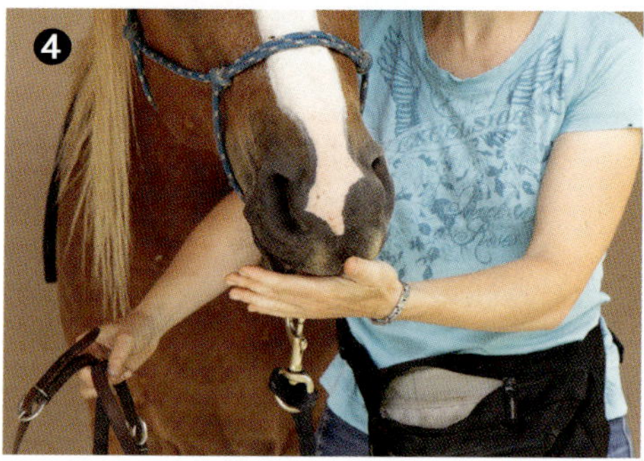

By removing the bit and deliberately allowing it to lightly impact the incisors on the way before you click and reward, you'll help the horse get used to the feeling of metal scraping against his teeth.

Step 1: The horse touches the bit with his lips on his own initiative; click and reward him.
Step 3: The horse grabs the bit, or you introduce it to him; click and reward him.
Step 4: Insert the bit farther into his mouth.
Reward each step by removing the bit each time.

Common Mistakes

- Removing the bit as soon as the horse tries to spit it out.

On the day actual dental care is scheduled, for an inexperienced horse, you can ask the vet or dental technician to carry out the dental work in several installments—they can complete a procedure or two, and then the horse can have a break and go back to his friends for a bit before the next procedure starts. If you notice that your horse is really getting agitated, you can ask to end the dental work for the day, or for sedation. If the work isn't finished yet, that's too bad. You can try again on another day, or start a session with mild sedation from the beginning. If certain kinds of dental equipment are in place and the horse is trying to rear or escape from you, he could seriously injure himself—and potentially you, too.

Review the signs of impatience in horses, because they're common during dental work that takes too long (see page 25). If you see these signs in your horse, you need to stop the treatment and give him a break. Otherwise, he'll escalate, and he, you, and the dental professional will all be in danger. Think about how you feel when you have to hold your mouth open for a long time at the dentist's. Having a moment to close your jaw and swallow before you continue is necessary, now and then.

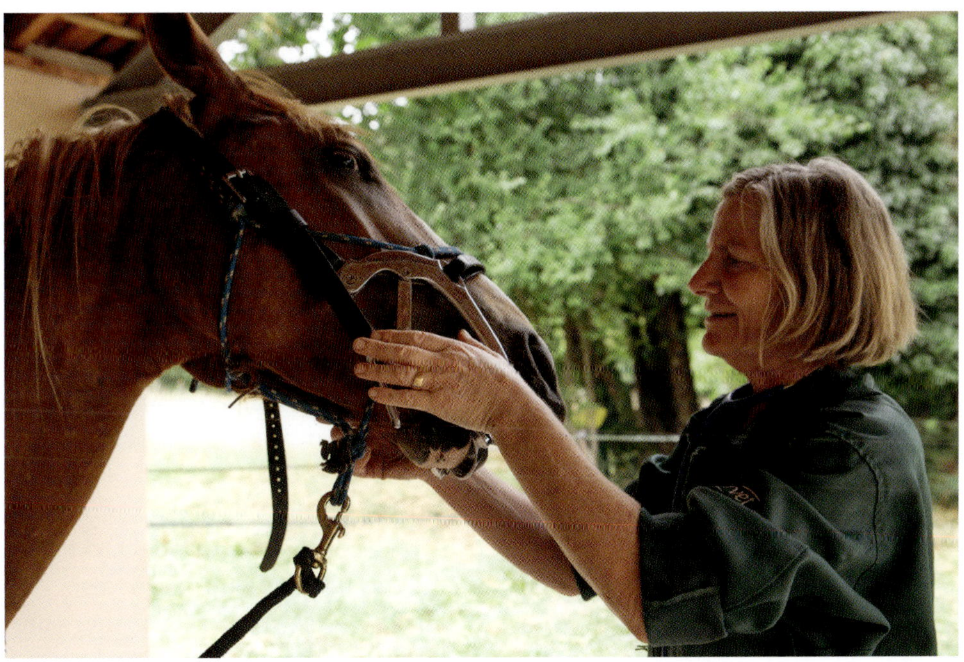

If your horse is not sedated, then it's a good idea to plan to take breaks and remove all equipment from his mouth to give his jaw joint a break. In this horse, you can see a wide-open eye with the white visible, and ears that are facing backward—signs of distress.

Using an Inhaler or Nebulizer

What's the Point?

Horses and ponies often suffer from respiratory problems (I can't say the same for certain about donkeys, because I don't have the data to back it up). Studies[61] report that 60 to 80% of horses are affected in a mild to moderate manner—they may not show clinical signs of respiratory issues at rest, but during exercise, they cough, experience shortness of breath, or otherwise have poor respiratory performance. A much smaller percentage of horses have severe problems, where they show respiratory distress at rest. These problems usually start out occasional and mild, and then evolve into asthma characterized by difficulty breathing in certain environmental conditions (surrounded by poor-quality hay, kept in a building with poor ventilation). Horses need inhalers in pretty much the same circumstances a human might:

- To treat inflammation of the respiratory tract (administering essential oils or corticosteroids);

- To relieve an acute, moderate attack (administering a bronchodilator or corticosteroids);

- As preventative care (for sports horses and racing horses with heavily stressed respiratory tracts).

Distribution of any product put into a nebulizer through the respiratory tract depends on all kinds of factors, including the size of the particles (which itself depends on the quality and technology used in the nebulizer), the nature of the product (whether it's water-based or oil-based), how deeply the horse is breathing, and how far the horse's airways are able to open. This last factor is directly linked to the horse's emotional state—a relaxed horse will take slower, deeper breaths than a tense or stressed horse, and medication administered through a nebulizer will be more effective. So it's very useful to train your horse to accept these objects, and to make sure they're used in a calm environment.*

What You Want the Horse to Do

- Stand still and breathe into a device without worry.

✦ What You Do

You might encounter any of three different types of equipment:

- An inhalation chamber, used for babies (a "babyhaler"), which covers one nostril with a silicone cup.

- A nasal spray, to be used on one nostril, disposable—train for this the same way as for the babyhaler.

- A nebulizer or inhaler, which is an electrical device. It includes a mask that covers the lower half of the horse's face, including his mouth, with a compressor connected to it by tubing; the compressor also makes noise. These days, there are

---

* Text written in consultation with Dr. Julie Dauvilier, a French professional veterinarian in equine internal medicine and equine sports medicine.

 —— PREPARING YOUR HORSE OR DONKEY FOR VETERINARY CARE

also ultrasonic and battery-powered nebulizers and inhalers that don't need the external compressor and don't have tubing. A single mask covers both nostrils.

If you're training your horse for a babyhaler or a nasal spray, you can work on this exercise anywhere. With a nebulizer or inhaler, you may need to find a place where you can plug in the device, depending on the model, and you'll also need somewhere you can position it so the horse won't trip over it or knock it over. If you don't have a helper available, you'll need to tie the horse for this.

✦ Step by Step: Babyhaler or Nasal Spray, with the Clicker and Approach-Retreat

Follow the same steps as for the Clipping exercise, either with approach-retreat, the combination of the clicker and approach-retreat, or even voluntary contact (see page 76), with the babyhaler or nasal spray container as the target you're asking the horse to touch.

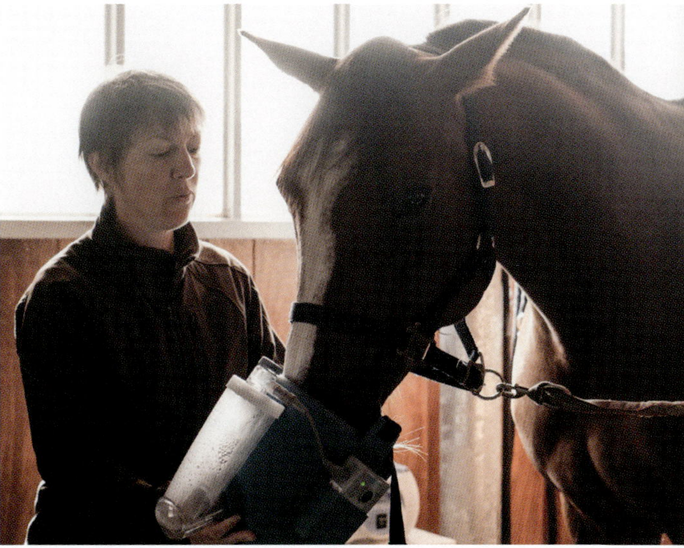

There are different devices out there, including models with batteries and no tubing. Training the horse to put his nose inside one on his own, as this horse is doing, will help him stay relaxed during their use.

The noise of the sprayer might not be very loud, depending on the spray bottle, but it's a good idea to train your horse to accept it anyway, to make sure he won't be startled and step away (see page 105).

Use a word or phrase ("Look out!", for example) before you squeeze the nasal spray's trigger to warn the horse something is coming; he'll be less surprised.[62]

With a combination of clicker techniques and targeting, you'll be asking your horse to voluntarily put his nose against the cup of the babyhaler.

1. Stand facing the horse on the same side as the nostril you want to use the babyhaler or nasal spray on. Present him with the object, and click when he touches it with his nose; reward him.

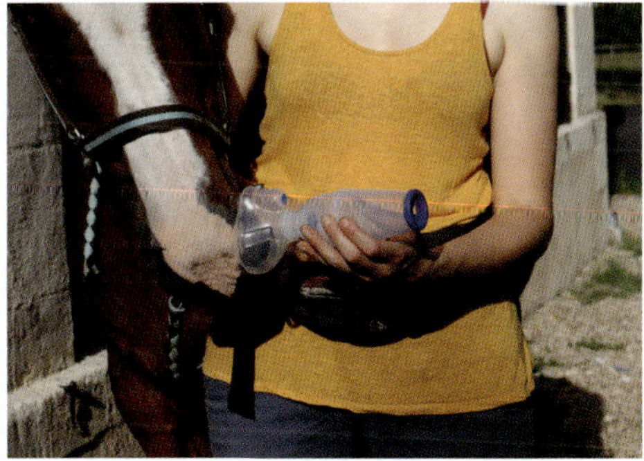

Here, this mare comes and puts her nose into the cup; after this, she'll be rewarded.

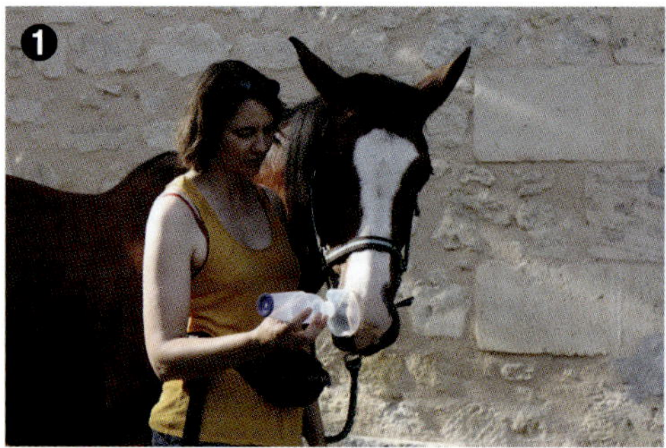

Step 2: The mare places her nose in the cup herself.

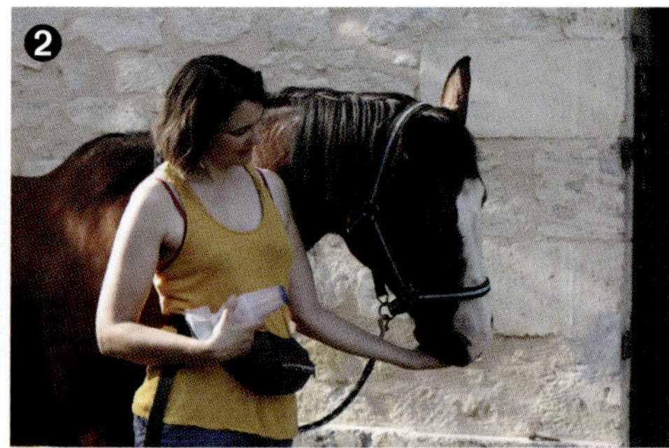

Reward each step along the way.

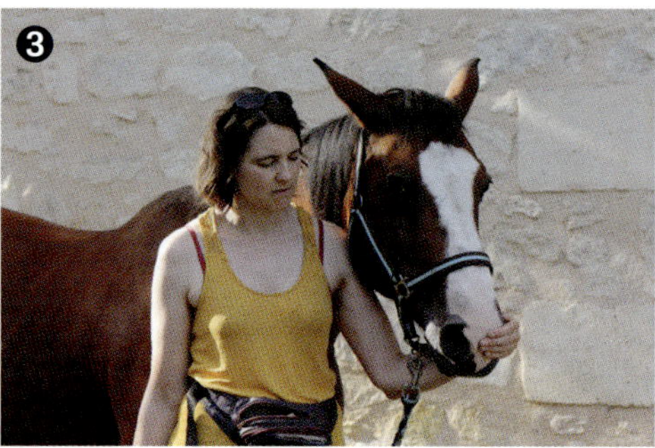

Step 6: Cover one nostril, blocking it.

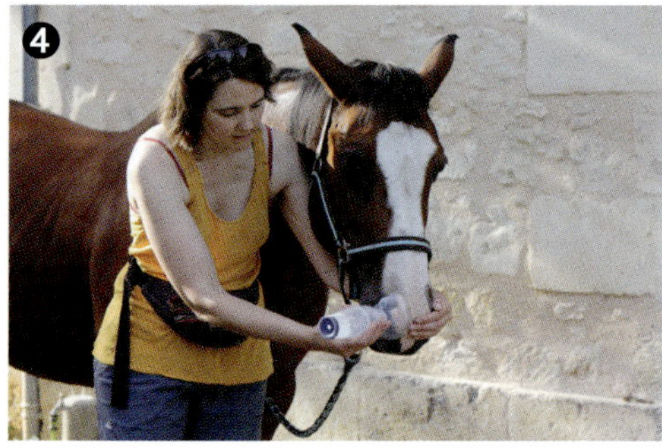

Step 7: Combine the results of step 2 and step 6!

2. Ask for more precision, until the horse has to touch the object with his nostril to get a click and a reward.

3. Increase the duration of the contact, waiting 2 seconds before clicking and rewarding the horse.

4. Click when the horse inhales while he's touching the object with his nostril; then move the object aside and reward him.

5. When he's succeeded at step 4 several times, move to his other side and repeat. It's better to work like this than to try to train from in front of your horse, because if you've already taught him the Statue, he might get confused and try to offer you stillness instead of a touch.

6. Have the horse touch the object with one nostril, block the other nostril, and wait for him to inhale; click when he does, uncover his nostrils, and reward him.

7. Go through the entire procedure fully; click and reward.

8. End the session on one of the first few steps, something easy such as presenting the object to the horse and having him touch it briefly with his nose.

9. After this, both of you will be prepared for you to actually use a

 — PREPARING YOUR HORSE OR DONKEY FOR VETERINARY CARE

medication cartridge in a device and release a puff into his nose. You can use a signal of encouragement to ask your horse to stick with it through several deep breaths without interrupting the procedure to reward him (see page 90). It'll take at least three or four breaths for the medication in one squeeze of the cartridge to move through the horse's respiratory system fully, and most cartridges will have around 12 squeezes to administer.

It's a good idea to split this training up across multiple sessions, either over the course of several days, or on the same day if treating the horse is a matter of urgency. Just remember that making sure the horse is relaxed will make this kind of medication more effective; it's worth it to take your time.

◆ Step by Step: Familiarizing the Horse with the Noise of a Nebulizer

Follow the same steps as for adjusting the horse to noise in the Clipping exercise (see page 93). With your horse tied a good distance away from the compressor:

1. Turn on the compressor;

2. Bring the horse a bucket of food (or a few carrots or something else he likes);

3. Return to the compressor while he eats, and make sure you shut it off before he's finished;

4. Repeat, several days in a row.

You should start to notice your horse waiting for his food to arrive when he hears the compressor start up, instead of worrying about it.

If your horse is too nervous about the noise to eat, move the compressor farther away, or tie your horse farther from it, until he's willing to eat while it's running.

After several sessions like this where your horse eats calmly:

1. Bring the compressor gradually closer to the horse, until it's in about the same position relative to him as it will be when the nebulizer is in use.

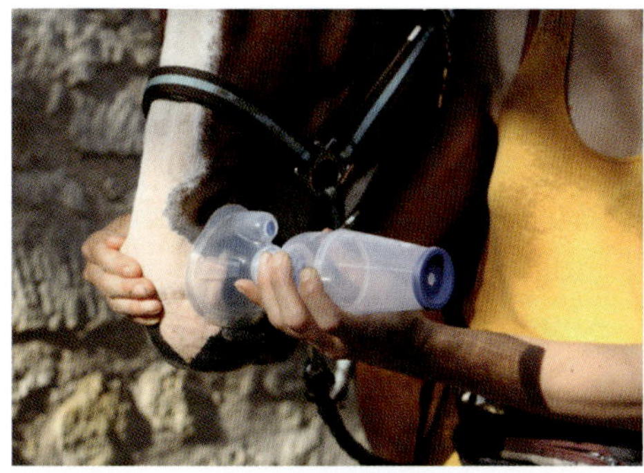

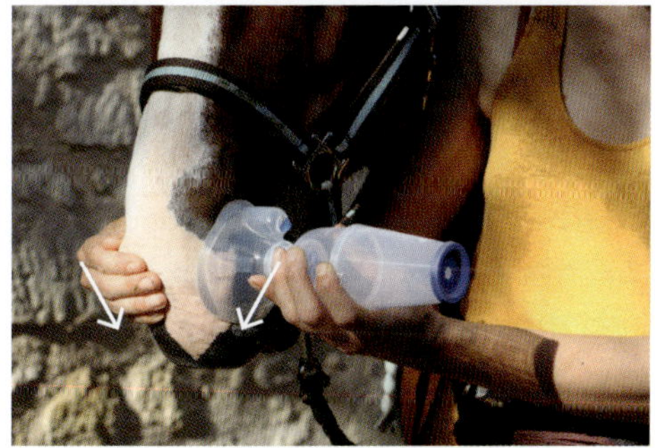

You'll have to pay attention and notice when your horse is inhaling so you can click at the right moment and teach him to take nice deep breaths. Look at the photo on the bottom, and you'll see the way the horse's nostrils have widened with his inhale just above the person's hand and the cup of the babyhaler, compared to the photo on the top.

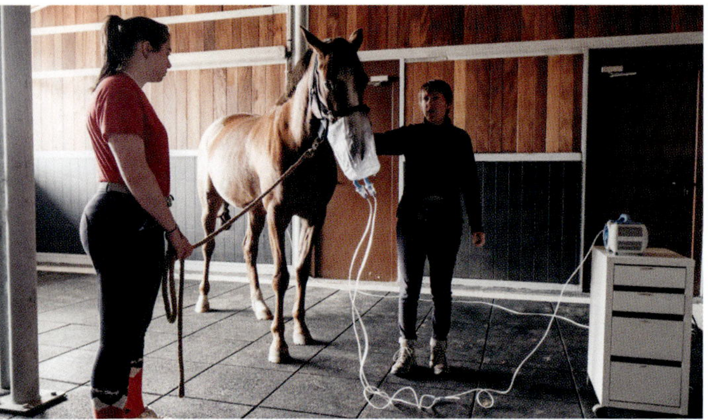

The movement of the tubes that run from an inhaler or nebulizer mask to the compressor when a horse moves his head may make him nervous. So it's a good idea to click and reward him when he stays still; he'll move his head less, which will make the tubes move less, too.

2. Repeat the same steps at each new distance.

Common Mistakes

- Shutting the compressor off when the horse is moving, instead of while he's still eating.

✦ Step by Step: Nebulizer or Inhaler Mask with the Clicker and Approach-Retreat

Before you actually start using an equine nebulizer or inhaler, you also need to teach your horse to accept the mask of it on his face. You can use approach-retreat by itself, but I'd recommend including clicks and food rewards:

1. Ask the horse to touch the mask with his nose without trying to put it on him, and reward him (see Touch-Click on page 47).

2. Ask the horse to touch the mask and hold it in place against his face without putting the strap behind his ears; wait for him to hold his head still, and when he does, click and immediately remove the mask, then reward him.

3. Repeat the previous step until you can put the mask up to his face and keep it there as easily as you can the noseband of a halter.

4. Put the mask on the horse again, and this time, pass the strap behind his ears—only for a second—before taking it off.

5. Put the mask on the horse and the strap behind his ears, and leave it there for a few seconds before taking it off.

6. Keep increasing the duration the horse is spending with the mask in place, alternating between longer durations and short ones.

Once the mask is staying in place on the horse longer, you can wait up to ten seconds before clicking, taking it off of him, and rewarding him.

✦ Step by Step: Nebulizer or Inhaler Medication with the Clicker and Approach-Retreat

Using both the clicker and the approach-retreat technique:

1. Plug the device in and hold the mask, with water in place of medication, approximately 6 feet away from the horse, facing him. Start the compressor. A

cloud of mist will come out. If the horse sees it, click and reward him without moving the mask closer to him (you can have a helper reward him when you click).

2. Repeat three more times, if the horse is calm. If he seems alert (he isn't blinking, or he's snorting, stepping away, tensing his neck, or raising and lowering his head to try to get a good look at the mist), move the mask away from him, and repeat a few more times until he's at ease.

3. Take a step closer, warn him something's about to happen, show him the mist or blow it up into a cloud, and if he doesn't move, click and reward him.

4. Repeat three more times.

5. Come closer to the horse, close enough for him to touch the mask easily if he chooses to do it, and if he touches it before the mist puffs out, click and reward him, and then click and reward him again when the mist does appear, even if he backs up. If he does back up, take a step away, wait for another cloud of mist, and click and reward him until he's willing to stand still again; then step closer.

6. Wait through several puffs, and see whether the horse stays still; if he does, click and reward him.

◆ Step by Step: Putting It All Together with the Clicker and Approach-Retreat

Turn on the compressor, and ask your horse to let you put the mask on him.

1. Once the mask is in place, give him a signal of encouragement (see page 90) to tell him he's

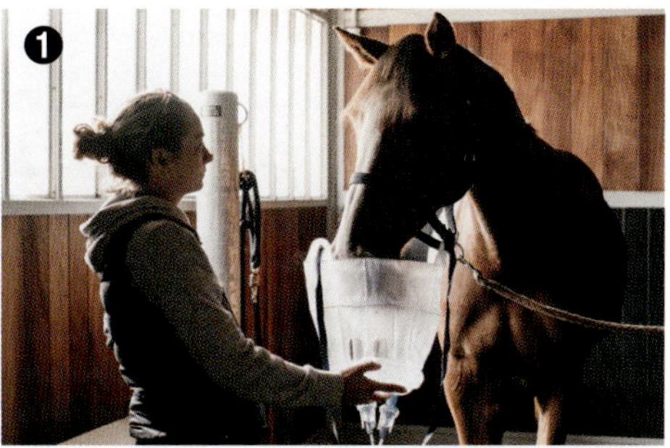

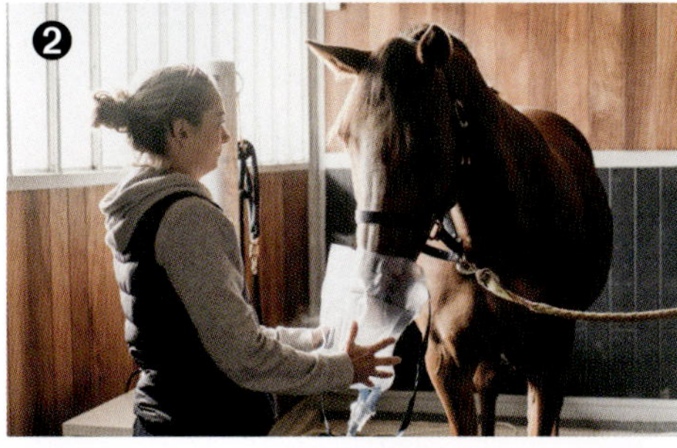

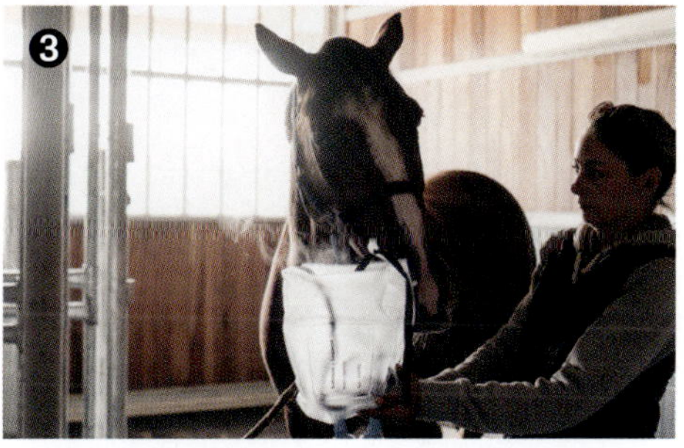

After learning to touch the mask voluntarily, this mare is willing to hold her nose above it ❶, and then to lower the end of her nose into it ❷. If she lowers her head into it even further, that's worth a click and a reward. The trainer is holding the mask, which keeps producing puffs of mist ❸ and she's going to reward the mare for standing still even if she takes her face out of the mask a couple times. This is another step you should take your time with.

doing the right thing by staying still. If the mask you have has holes in the bottom, as some of them do, you can click and slide small rewards in for the horse. Depending on the situation, he might have to keep the mask on for up to 30 minutes; if you can take it off intermittently, then go ahead and give him breaks, and reward him.

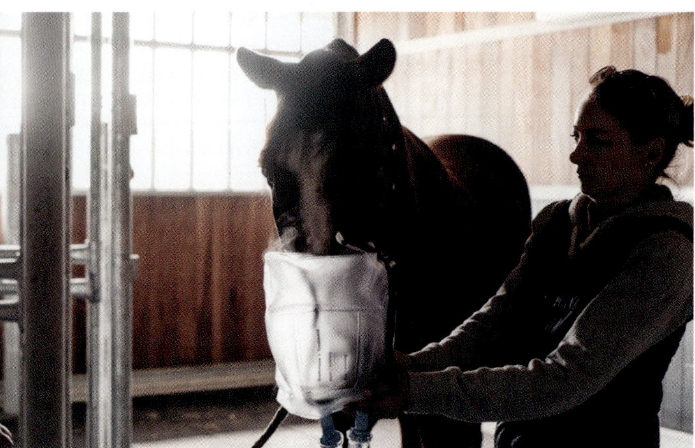

This mare willingly puts her nose in the mask while the compressor is running and mist is puffing out.

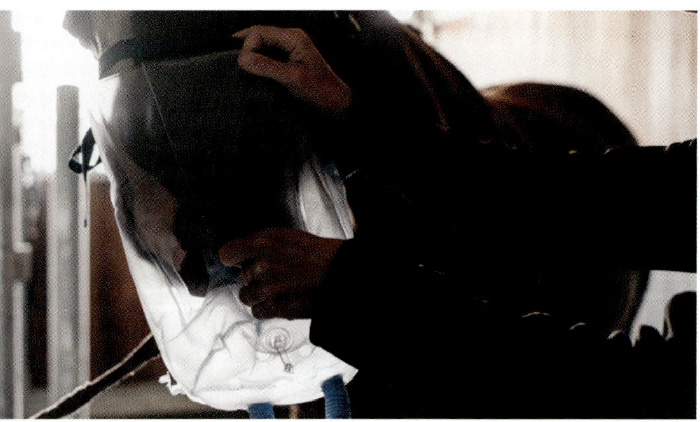

With some masks, you can pass rewards through holes in the bottom during a long session with the nebulizer or inhaler.

2. At the end of his session with the inhaler or nebulizer, ask him for something very simple and give him lots of rewards for it, or a special reward he really loves.

Horses in serious respiratory distress will usually feel the medication providing them some relief and relax, even with the mask on. For horses who don't feel it, or are too distracted by the mask and their own impatience to feel it, you may need to try multiple shorter sessions instead of one long treatment to administer the full dose of medication. It's always better to relieve your horse's frustrations than to end up teaching him to hate having the mask on. You'll be able to tell when your horse needs a break by his behavior (see page 25 for some signs to look out for).

Common Mistakes

- Taking the mask off when the horse moves. Some horses need a moment to discover they can still breathe with the mask on—give your horse time and see whether he calms down.

 — PREPARING YOUR HORSE OR DONKEY FOR VETERINARY CARE

Performing an Injection or Drawing Blood

What's the Point?

An injection—a shot—is used to administer something beneath the skin, into a muscle, or into a vein. What might that something be?

- Vaccines;
- Antibiotics;
- Anti-inflammatory medications (after an operation, to treat lameness, and so on);
- Tranquilizers (to make examination or treatment easier).

A blood test with a sample taken from the jugular vein will feel about the same as an injection to the horse, even though in this case the veterinarian is taking blood, not injecting anything.

Most injections will probably be done by a vet, but with a prescription medication the horse needs to take over the long term, a vet may ask the horse's owner to perform them.

What You Want the Horse to Do

- Stand still, with the head raised.

What You'll Need

- An empty syringe, or a pen cap or pencil to simulate the touch of a needle.
- If you want to train your horse to accept a brief piercing of his skin, ask your vet for a very fine needle, and make sure to disinfect both the needle and the area of the horse's body you plan to practice on before you start.

- A given, but: a clicker and food rewards your horse likes.

◆ What You Do

You shouldn't tie your horse for this exercise, if you can avoid it. You can work alone, with a halter and a lead rope, or you can ask someone to help you (standing on the same side of the horse as you are, and helping to limit his movements); you can also work alone with the horse at liberty, if you've already practiced other exercises this way and your horse is responsive to your signals and requests (see the Clipping exercise on page 93 for reminders about safety if the horse is on a lead rope).

When it comes to the procedure itself, the specific area where you need to perform the injection and the

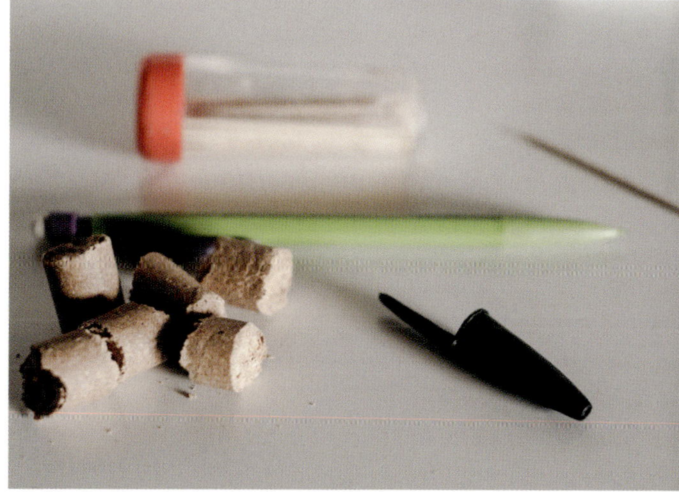

You don't need to be a professional vet to train your horse to accept injections and blood draws; you can simulate the sensations with ordinary objects that have points.

way you're supposed to do it, your vet will show you what you need to know.

The training as I've laid it out here does not simulate specific kinds of injections in detail (for example, some medications have to be injected slowly, because they're viscous and a rapid injection would be painful).

✦ Step by Step: Approach-Retreat

One method of restraint is to take a fold of skin in your hand (see page 66). Doing that exercise first is useful here; adding a simulated injection onto the end will be nothing but a formality. Here are the key steps:

- Approach the horse and touch his neck.
- As soon as he stands still, stop touching him and move away.
- Gradually increase the amount of contact you have with his neck, waiting for him to stand still, and then lift your hand away and step back.

Not every kind of injection starts with taking a fold of skin; it's a consistent first step for *subcutaneous* injections (where the medication needs to go under the skin).

1. Touch the horse with your hand flat, while he's standing still.

2. Take a fold of skin between your thumb and fingers for a second; repeat until the horse stays still through two repetitions in a row.

3. Increase the duration you're holding that fold of skin from two to four seconds.

4. Make the contact a little less comfortable (take a firmer hold of the skin).

5. Pinch the skin, and press next to the part you're pinching with the tip of your pen cap, pencil, or other pointy object.

6. It might feel mean, but make sure you're giving the horse a real prick with the object—remember, you're trying to prepare him for the feeling of a vet piercing his skin with a needle.

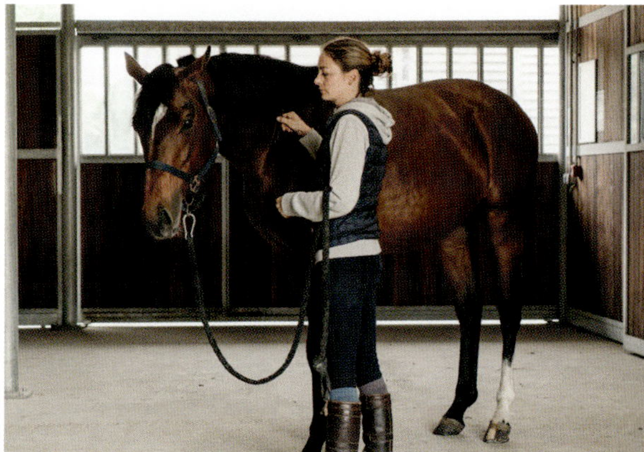

The first few times you do each of these steps, the horse might raise his head. Wait until he stops lifting it and is holding still to release the fold of skin; after a few more repetitions, wait until he's lowered his head again before you let go.

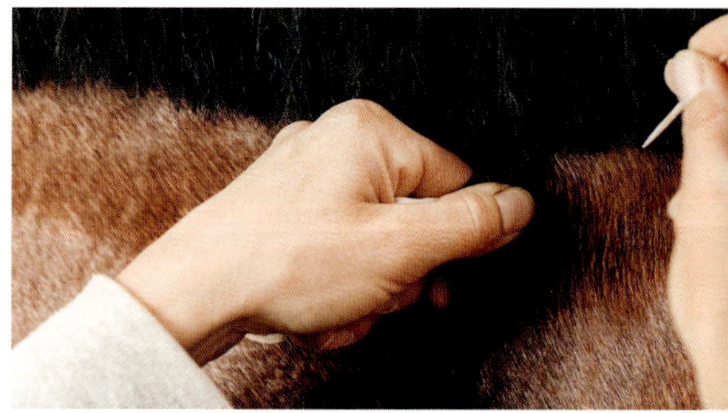

Step 5: taking a fold of skin and simulating the poke of a needle with a toothpick.

Learning from Experience

In a video you might have seen crossing your social media feeds (scan the QR code to watch it now), injection shyness is solved in a total of 1 minute and 16 seconds by Gemma Pearson, equine behavior specialist, during a 9-sequence approach-and-retreat session. The horse initially shows avoidance reactions when approached—he throws his head up, steps back, moves forward, tries to push with his head, turns his hindquarters toward his handler, and then shakes his head back and forth during the exercise and raises a foreleg. After the fifth time a fold of his skin is taken, though, he's willing to stand still. The handler is then able to move closer to the horse and stand in front of him, and the trainer can let go of his halter with her left hand, use that hand to take another fold of skin, and simulate an injection with her right hand before actually performing it.*

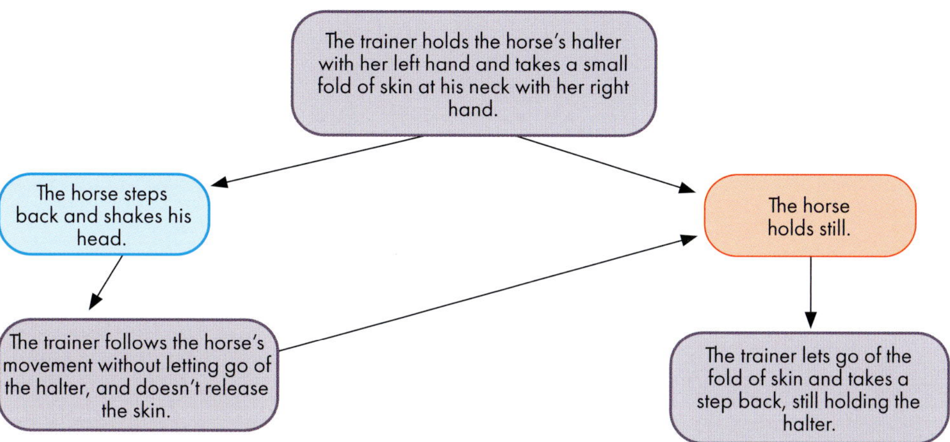

Step 2 in detail, as it plays out in the video described above.

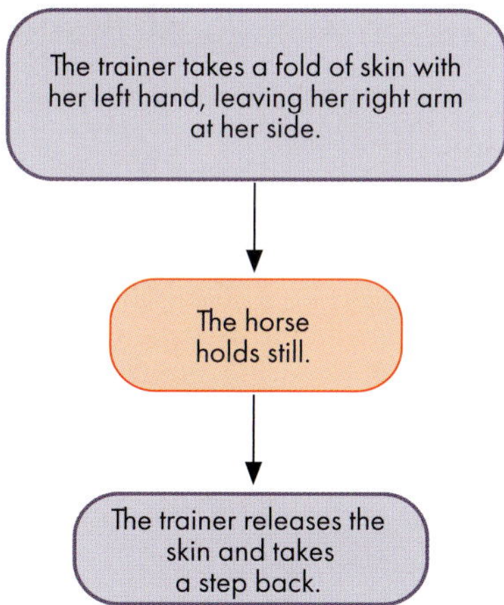

Step 3 in detail, with these happening two at a time, as they play out in the video described above.

* Pearson Gemma, 2015. "Practical application of equine learning theory, part 2," *In Practice*, Volume 37, pages 286-292, doi:10.1136/inp.h2483.

- Breaking off contact (whether by releasing the fold of skin or by lifting the object away, depending on the step you're on) when the horse moves. You have to follow his movement until he stops—not trapping him, just staying with him so his movement can't bring the contact to an end.
- Asking the horse to hold still for too long. Settle for one second, at first, and gradually increase to three or four seconds.

✦ Step by Step: The Clicker and Approach-Retreat

The exercise that teaches you to take a fold of skin in your hand (see page 66) is useful here, especially since it uses the clicker also; adding a simulated injection onto the end will be nothing but a formality. Here are the key steps:

1. Touch the horse's neck with your hand flat.

2. Take a small fold of skin between your thumb and fingers.

3. Take a fold of skin with a firmer grip.

4. Increase the duration you're holding that fold of skin for.

5. Take a fold of skin, and then bring your other hand (the one holding the clicker) toward the horse also.

6. Increase the duration you're holding that fold of skin for with your other hand beside it.

7. Grasp your pen cap, pencil, or other pointy object with the hand

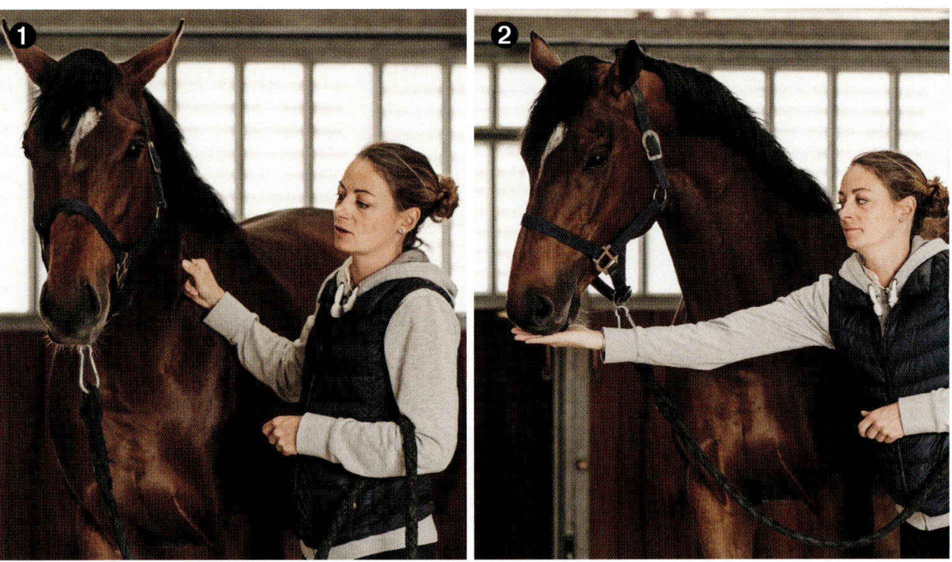

The horse stands still when the trainer takes a fold of skin in her hand ❶; the trainer clicks her tongue, and then rewards him ❷. This is step 2 using *clicker training*.

holding the clicker, while your arm is at your side, and then approach the horse again to take a fold of skin—just holding the pointy object, so it isn't touching the horse but the horse can see that there's something in your hand.

8. Take a fold of skin and press the pointy object into the skin right next to it.

9. Repeat step 8 for a longer duration.

10. Repeat step 8, applying more pressure with the object.

11. Repeat the entire exercise from the beginning, but with another person near the horse—starting with touching the horse's neck with your hand held flat, and then taking a small fold of skin, taking it more firmly, taking it while you have the object in your other hand, and taking it and pressing the object into the skin beside it.

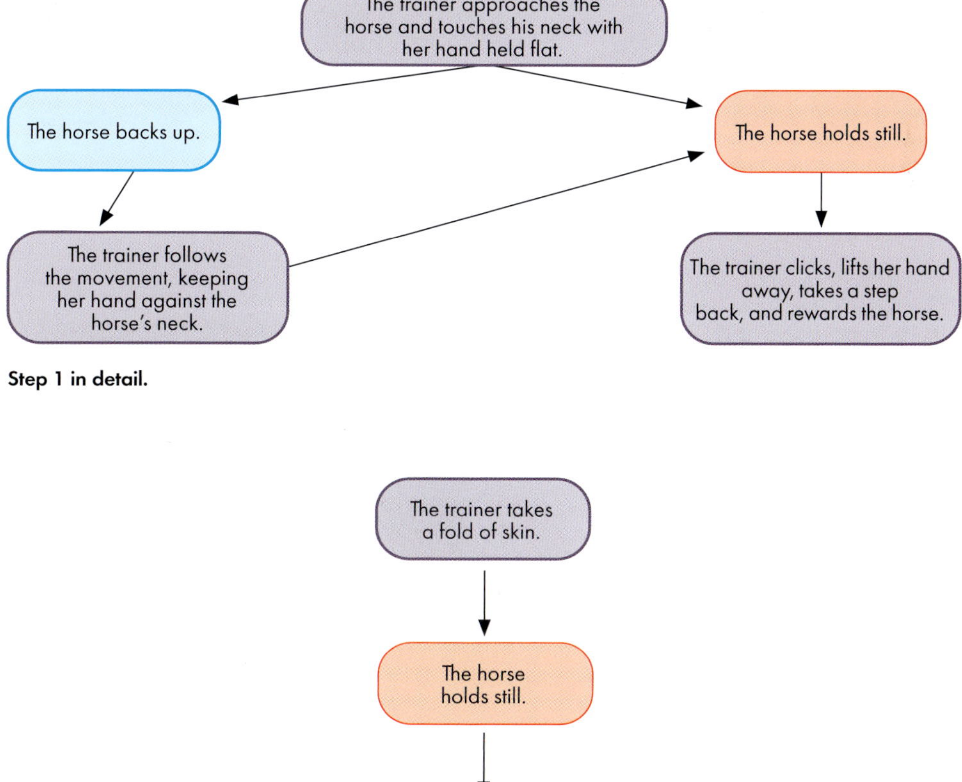

Step 1 in detail.

Step 2 in detail.

Learning from Experience

Working with a horse who reacted defensively to injections, Gemma Pearson, an equine education professional in the UK, reached every milestone in this exercise with 22 click-reward cycles, in 4 minutes and 50 seconds. The horse's halter was held by a handler; the horse started out showing avoidance responses. You can watch the video of this demonstration, part of the "Don't Break Your Vet!" series on YouTube, titled "Easy Injections" (scan the QR code to go straight to it).

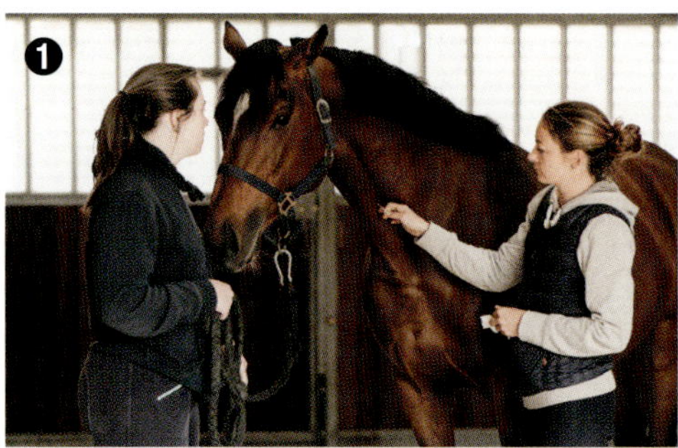

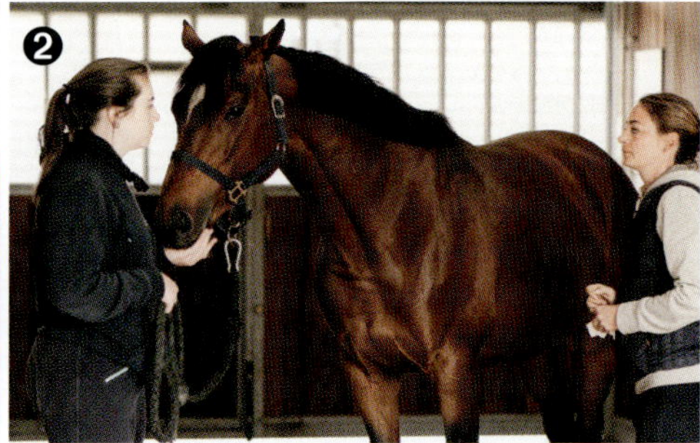

The procedure here is essentially the same as the steps in the exercise I describe, except the trainer isn't taking a fold of skin. This is the final step: with another person beside the horse, the trainer simulates an injection or a blood draw with the poke of a toothpick ❶. After clicking, the trainer stepped away, and the handler gave the horse his reward ❷.

For horses who really don't like injections, you might want to simulate the process in even more detail:

1. Take out a square of cotton gauze.

2. Apply disinfectant to it.

3. Let the horse see the syringe.

4. Push a little water out of the syringe.

5. Approach the horse with the cotton ball and syringe in your hands.

6. Tap his neck with your fingertips (vets often do this before an intramuscular injection).

7. Press on his jugular vein (this will happen during an intravenous injection or blood draw).

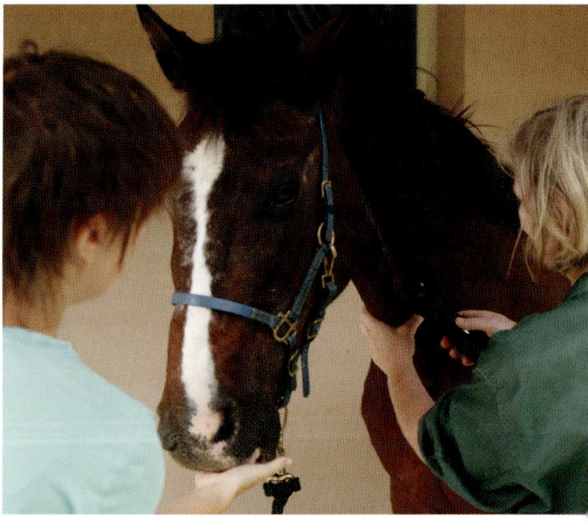

Clipping the horse's neck so the vet can see the jugular vein better might be necessary before a blood draw or intravenosus injection. Here, you can see this horse's upper eyelid lowering—he's relaxed as he accepts his reward while being clipped.

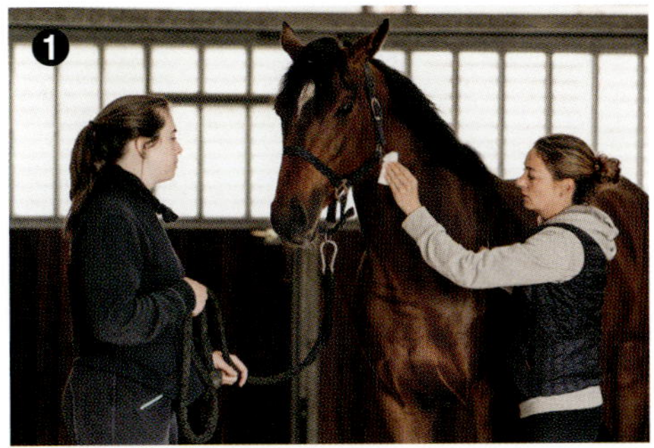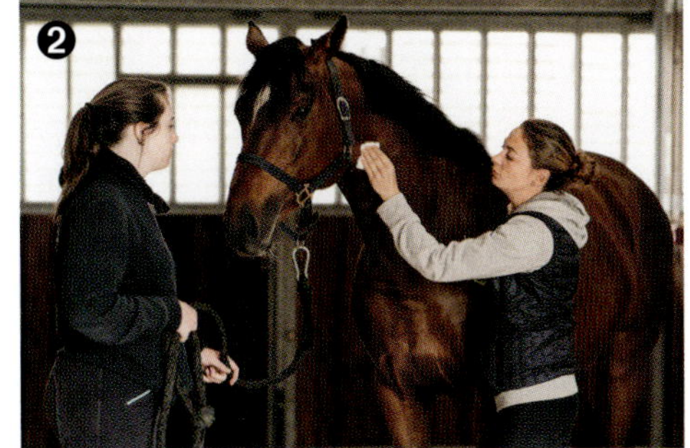

You can see from the expression on this horse's face that he's a little worried: his head is raised, his eyes are wide open, his ears are out to the side and facing downward, and his mouth is tight. He's wary of the cotton gauze being used to swab disinfectant on his jugular vein ❶. But he starts to relax slightly, lowering his head, as the training continues ❷.

8. Practice any other action you or the vet might perform!

All of these actions and sensations will be consistently associated with a reward for the horse.

Here's how to proceed:

1. Do something the horse doesn't like—for example, approach him with a square of cotton gauze soaked in disinfectant, stopping as far away as you need to in order to avoid making him decide to back away. Take it slow, and see how close you can get without the horse moving.

2. Stay there, with your horse holding still.

3. Click and reward. Remember to set down the cotton before approaching the horse to reward him, if you're working alone, because otherwise you may trigger a fear response. If the horse is very alert, you can even throw his reward onto the ground in front of him instead of approaching him—that way, you don't risk him deciding to run away. You do have to make sure he's able to find his reward on the ground, though.

You'll know your horse is starting to associate veterinary procedures with rewards if you notice him anticipating the arrival of food—for example, as you're taking a syringe out of your pocket, he's paying attention and turning his nose toward you. This is a sign that his associations with the syringe are strong, and you can move on to another procedure he isn't as familiar with. Sue McDonnell, an equine behavior specialist, has concluded that even in the most difficult cases, 10 repetitions are enough to allow you to move on to the next step.

Once you have all the pieces in place, you need to put them together to mimic a complete veterinary procedure. Be aware that during the most painful or uncomfortable part—the moment a needle pierces the horse's skin, or the moment the injection is pushed through the needle—you might need to reward the horse a little more. You can save a treat he really likes for this moment, or give him more of the usual. To make this step even easier, ask your vet for a very thin needle and practice piercing your horse's skin with it, too.

Even after an injection has been performed with the horse completely calm throughout, you'll want to make sure he keeps his positive associations with the procedure.

Review this exercise without the unpleasant part (piercing the skin), using food rewards, a few days before the vet's going to come. If you practice it two or three times a year, you can review it the day before an actual injection is coming.

Common Mistakes

- Breaking off contact or stepping away when the horse moves.

- Clicking when the horse is backing up or raising his head.

- Asking the horse to hold still for too long without rewarding him for it.

- Taking this training for granted after an injection goes smoothly. To avoid this mistake, repeat the exercise another 10 times at least, with rewards, so your horse's most recent memory of the procedure isn't the vet piercing his skin for real with the needle. Ken Ramirez, who trains all kinds of wild mammals, recommends 100 "pretend" procedures for every 1 real procedure.[64] This ratio might

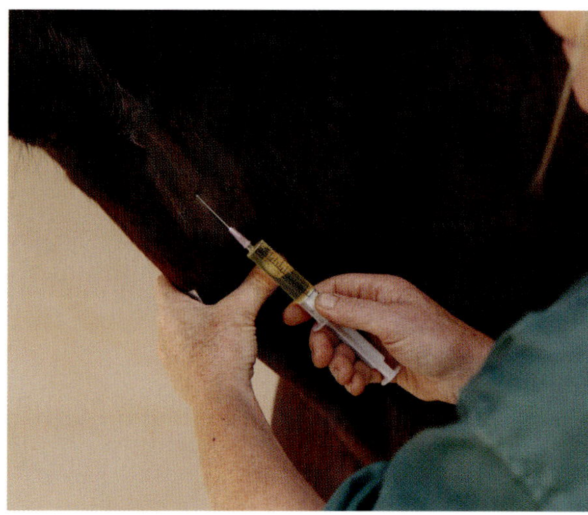

If you want to practice piercing the skin so your horse knows what to expect, make sure practice *without* piercing it more often, with food rewards each time.

seem ridiculous—and it probably isn't necessary for your horse, who isn't a wild animal. But if you do 10 sessions, spread out across a few days three times a year, and practice the final step with a reward 10 times in each session, suddenly you've done it 100 times. So it's not as unthinkable as it might sound!

- Refusing to reward your horse for standing still if the vet has missed the vein or isn't successful drawing blood. The horse has done *his* job, and he deserves that reward.

◆ Step by Step: The Clicker and the "Stop Button"

Ask the horse to stand still by giving him a target—your hand, for example—to press his nose against. While he's doing this, the vet can perform the injection or blood draw. However, making this work means:

- Preparing the horse by practicing with the target you're going to use (see the Touch-Click exercise on page 47);

- Familiarizing the horse with the overall procedure using clicker or approach-retreat techniques.

Why invest so much time and effort in this training? Because you're adding a new tool to your toolbox. This method is very good for particularly timid horses, ponies, and donkeys—not necessarily those who dislike injections a lot, but those who are nervous around strangers, including the vet.

Learning from Experience

During the photography session that gave us many of the photos for this book, Victor, my pony, kept withdrawing his nose from my palm when the vet lifted both of her hands to his neck to perform an injection. This told me we needed to stop and break the procedure down into smaller steps. We started with the vet touching his neck with one hand. When he was able to accept that, with several click-reward cycles, we were able to progress to simulating the injection with both of the vet's hands. The vet could tell, just by touching him with her fingers, that his blood pressure had dropped; he was relaxing. (That part, I would never have noticed.) Although Victor was still a little worried—you can see it in his face here—using the "stop button" technique let him alert me right away when he was uncomfortable, before he could get seriously stressed or afraid.

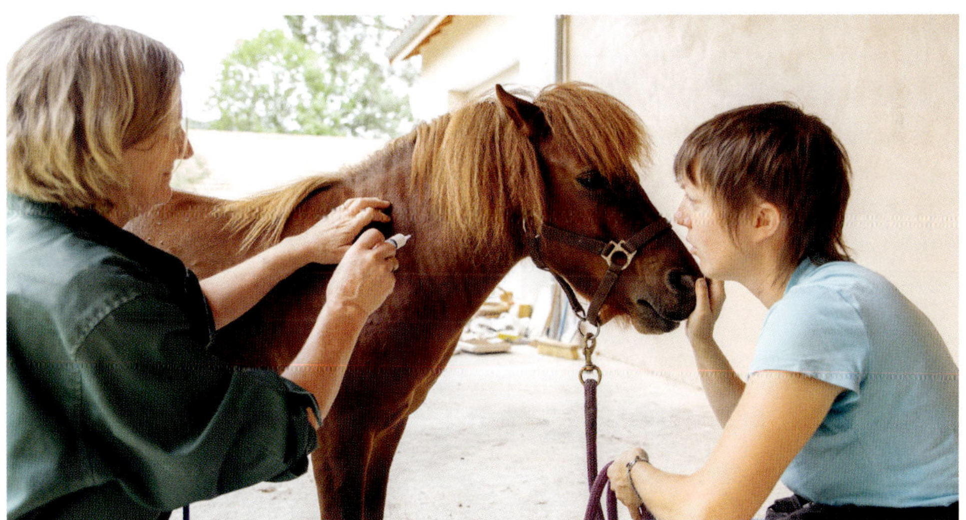

Victor signals his willingness to let the procedure continue by maintaining the contact of his nose against my palm, even though he's visibly worried (his head is raised slightly, his eyes are wide, and his ears are facing backward).

Deworming or Administering Medication Orally

What's the Point?

Teaching your horse to accept a syringe in his mouth will make it easier to:

- Deworm him regularly;

- Give him a liquid or paste supplement that doesn't have to be concealed in food (for overweight horses, it's good to be able to treat them without feed; for horses who are suspicious of any unusual smell in their food, or who aren't eating at all, the advantages are obvious);

- Administer oral tranquilizers, if you have no other option (or if your veterinarian has prescribed it).

What You Want the Horse to Do

- Willingly come into contact with the syringe;

- Hold his head still while you're inserting the syringe into his mouth.

What You'll Need

- An empty, clean oral syringe (to avoid lingering odors that might be associated with bad memories of past oral dewormers or pastes), or an empty injection syringe (the small tips on these, even without a needle, are less comfortable against the corner of the horse's mouth, but you can make this exercise work with them).

- A container of applesauce.

✦ What You Do: Approach-Retreat

If you've already trained your horse to accept being restrained by the halter

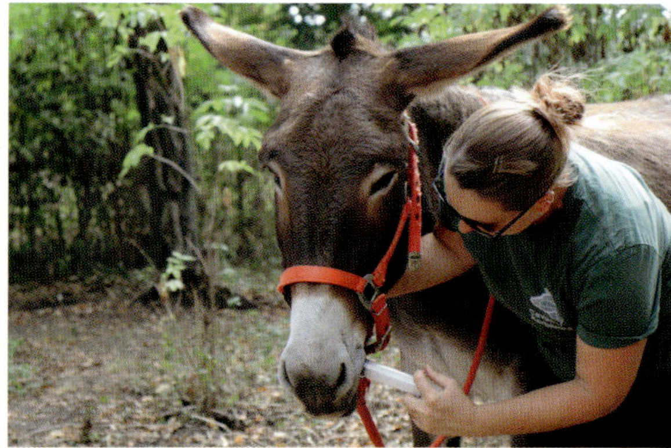

Being able to accept medications administered orally without stress will be a big help to your equine throughout his life.

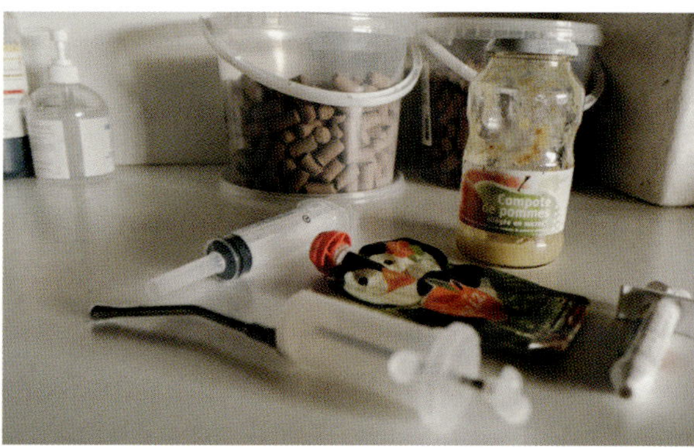

Here are several different tools that can help you with this exercise: there's an oral syringe in the foreground, an empty syringe of dewormer to the right, a syringe with a classic tip to the upper left, and a bottle that can be filled with applesauce.

(see Grasping the Halter Firmly on page 59), he'll be less likely to lift his head during this exercise. However, if time is short and you need to teach your horse this exercise as quickly as possible, you can start here, and go back to other exercises another time.

Your horse should be wearing his halter, with a lead rope attached. Position yourself at his shoulder to avoid taking a blow from his head if he decides to raise it suddenly. With the lead rope draped over his neck, hold his halter with one hand at the base of the noseband and hold the syringe in the other. Holding the halter while you do this will make it easier for you to follow your horse's motions and keep the syringe in his mouth until he settles.

- Hold the syringe near an area where the horse is comfortable with touch, and touch him with it.
- When the horse is standing still, move the syringe away.
- Repeat, gradually moving the syringe closer to the corner of the horse's mouth.

✦ Step by Step

1. Move the syringe toward the throatlatch.
2. Touch the cheek with it.
3. Touch the corner of the horse's mouth with it.
4. Touch the corner of the horse's mouth with it, and press in lightly.
5. Touch the corner of the horse's mouth with it, press lightly, and insert the end of the syringe at the corner of the mouth.
6. Repeat, pushing the syringe a little farther into the horse's mouth.

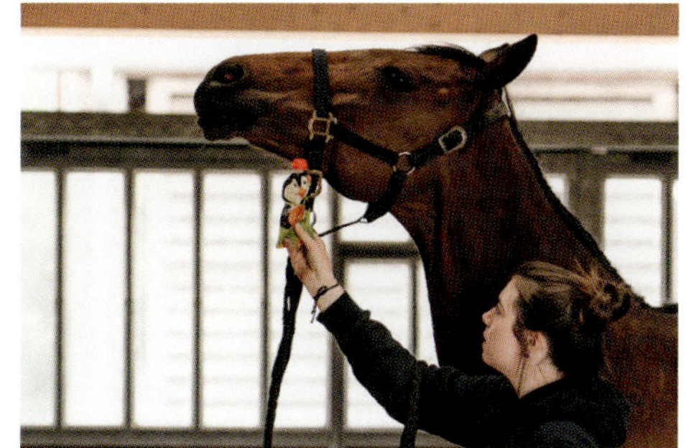

If your horse raises his head whenever you reach for his mouth, clicker training is a good way to teach him to accept it and cooperate with you.

7. Depress the plunger—you can fill your syringe with the applesauce, or, if you don't have a syringe available, you can follow these steps with the open top of the applesauce container, and then squeeze it to give the horse a taste.

Make sure you're pointing the syringe across the horse's mouth sideways or upward toward the back of it. If you point it down toward the front of his mouth, he might spit out whatever you're trying to give him.

Common Mistakes

- Breaking off contact if the horse moves (restraining the horse gently with a hand on his halter will help you avoid this pitfall).

Learning from Experience

Working with a mare who liked to raise her head to avoid deworming, Gemma Pearson, an equine education professional in the UK, achieved all the milestones in this exercise in 13 approach-retreat cycles. It took her 4 minutes and 15 seconds. You can find the demonstration video, part of the "Don't Break Your Vet!" series, titled, "Worry-Free Worming" (or scan the QR code to go straight to it).

Learning from Experience: In Pictures

This series of photos shows the key stages in this exercise, with several techniques combining to the trainer's advantage: light restraint at the noseband of the halter to limit the movement of the horse's head, approach-retreat with a bottle of applesauce and then with a syringe, and clicker training as reinforcement throughout. The horse, at the click of the trainer's tongue, knows the exact moment when he's done what he's supposed to do; the object touching him goes away, and he gets a reward, which motivates him to keep participating in the exercise. We bring a horse from resistance to cooperation in the space of a few minutes—but this training needs to be repeated at least a few times to make it stick.

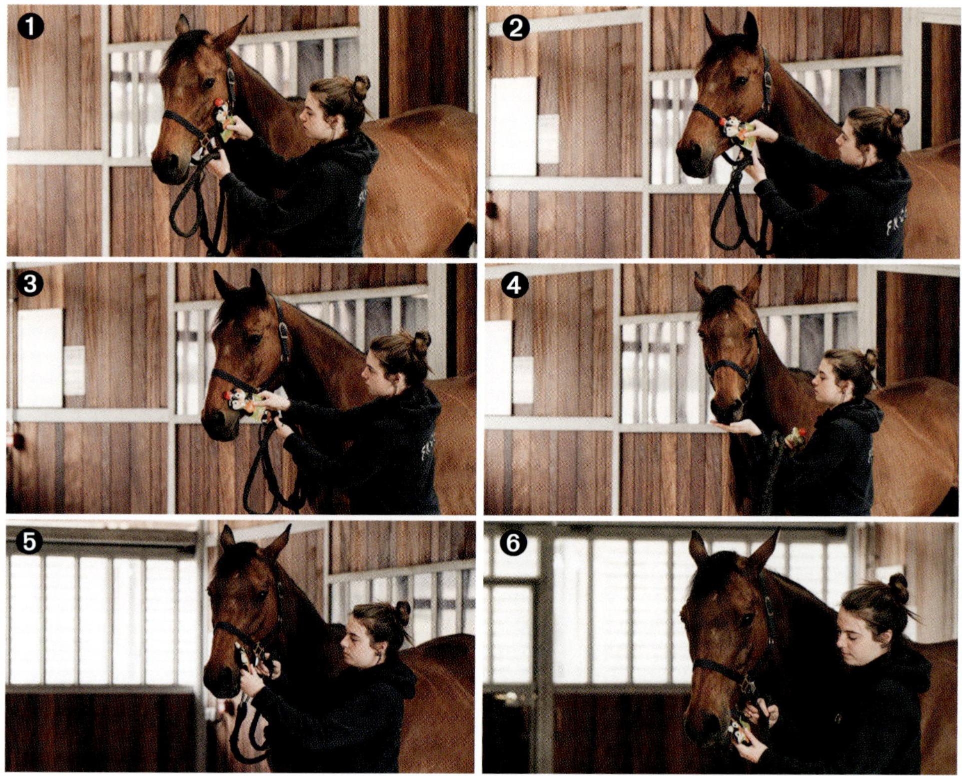

With a light amount of restraint, we touch the cheek ❶; we back up and start again without breaking off the contact if the horse raises his head ❷, moving down the cheek ❸, rewarding the horse at each step along the way ❹ as we continue to the corner of the mouth ❺. Keeping the contact brief, and breaking it off as soon as the horse is holding still, combined with the arrival of a food reward, leads the horse to begin to relax ❻.

- Moving from bottom to top—from the front of the lips to the corner of the mouth. Contact starting at the cheek and moving down is better, to avoid startling the horse with a touch he can't see coming.

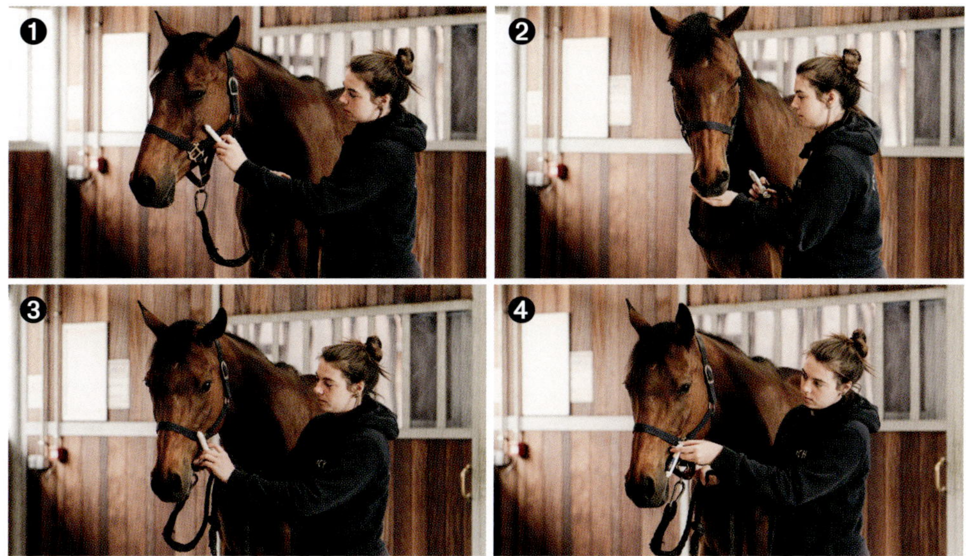

Another part of the same session as on the facing page, now with an empty dewormer syringe instead of a bottle of applesauce, but following the same progression. We need less restraint, or none at all ❶; we continue to reward each step along the way ❷. Notice the change in the horse's expression, compared to photo 1 on the facing page: his ears are facing forward more often ❸, and his head is lower ❹.

✦ What You Do: The Clicker and Voluntary Contact

To teach a horse to cooperate when you need to give him dewormer or another oral medication, you'll follow the same fundamental steps as for preparing him for eye care (see page 137). In this case, the target you'll ask him to touch is the syringe, not your hand. With this technique, the horse is the one who's responsible for maintaining contact, so it won't work well if the horse's head is restrained. You can work with the horse in a halter, with his lead rope draped over his neck, or you can work in "protected contact," with the horse in his stall and you outside of it, on the other side of the closed door. That way, you'll be safe from a strike with a foreleg.

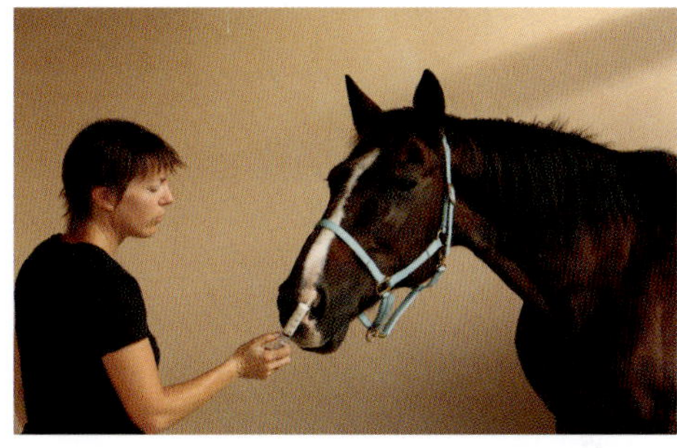

The horse will need to touch the syringe with his upper lip.

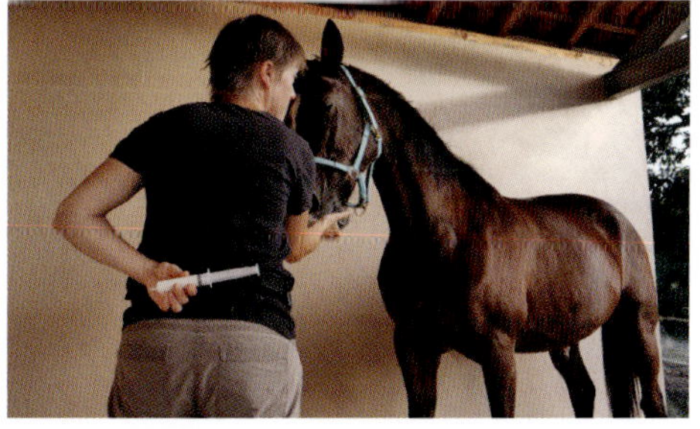

Hide the syringe behind your back when you click and reward the horse; otherwise, the horse might think he's supposed to touch it again and get confused.

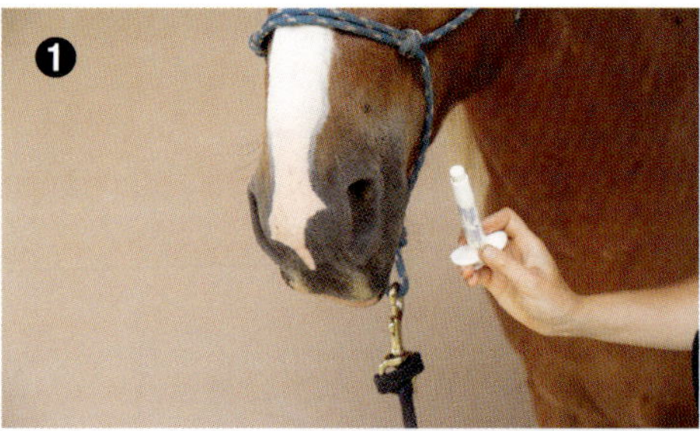

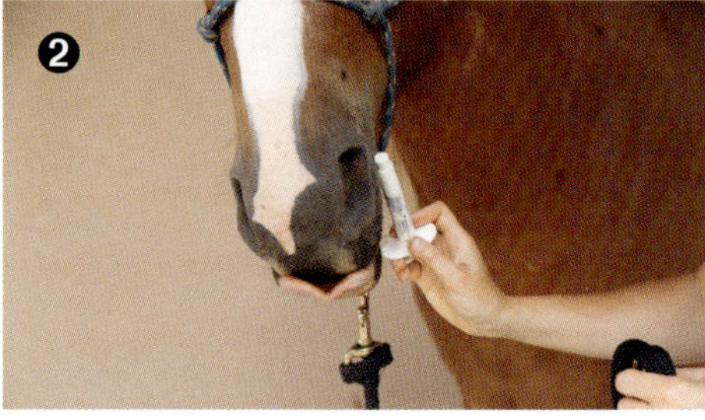

Step 2: I position the syringe and wait ❶; as soon as the horse touches the syringe, I click ❷.

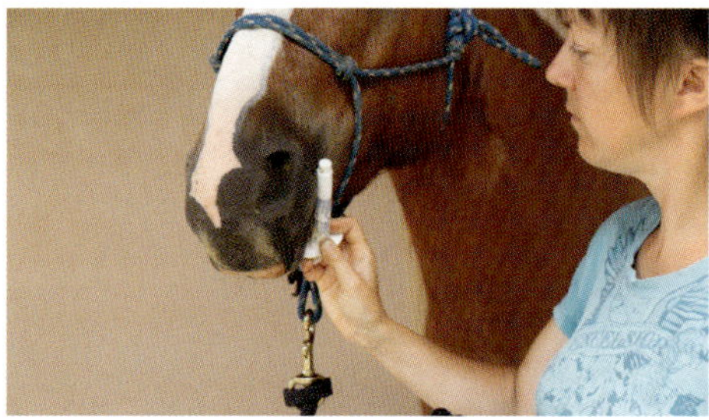

Step 5: Instead of clicking as soon as the horse touches the syringe, I wait one more second and then click, withdraw the syringe, and reward the horse.

Ask the horse to touch the syringe with his upper lip.
- Click.
- With the syringe behind your back, reward the horse with the other hand.

◆ Step by Step

1. Let the horse sniff the syringe; click, remove the syringe, and reward him.

2. Wait until he touches the syringe with his cheek; click, remove the syringe, and reward him.

3. Position the syringe at the back of the nostril nearest you; when the horse touches it with his face, click, remove the syringe, and reward him.

4. Position the syringe near the corner of the horse's mouth; when the horse touches it with his face, click, remove the syringe, and reward him.

5. Ask for two seconds of contact at the corner of the mouth; click, remove the syringe, and reward the horse.

6. Wait for the horse to touch the syringe at the corner of his mouth again and insert it just a little bit; click, remove the syringe, and reward him.

7. Repeat, inserting the syringe farther; click, remove the syringe, and reward the horse.

8. Insert the syringe far enough to administer the medication; click, remove the syringe, and reward the horse.

The idea is for the horse to be the one touching the syringe; in the end, he'll take it into his mouth himself. Offer the syringe to him vertically at first; once you get to the point where you're inserting it at the corner of his mouth, hold it at an angle, directing it toward the back of his mouth. If you hold it sideways (as if it were a bit), you might squeeze the medication out the other side, instead of into his mouth.

— **PREPARING YOUR HORSE OR DONKEY FOR VETERINARY CARE**

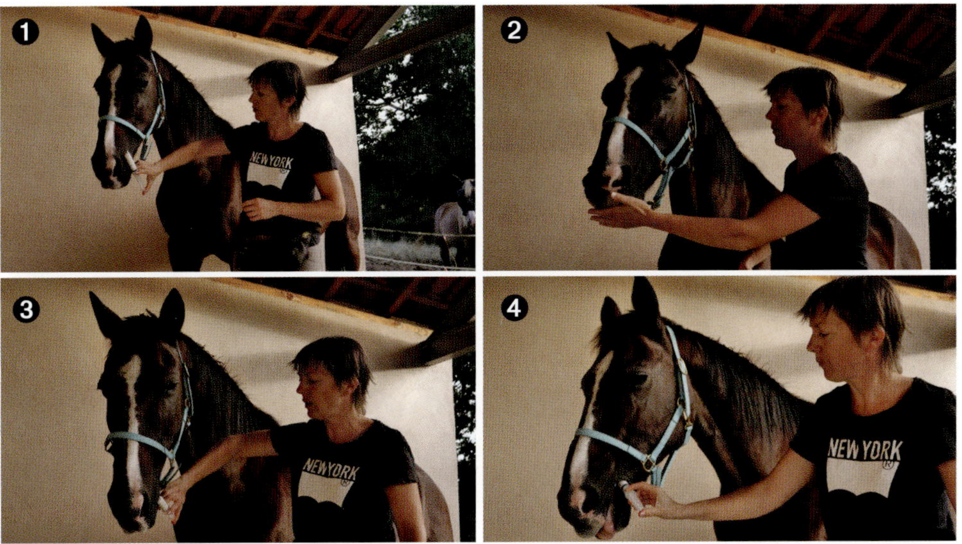

Position the syringe ❶, reward the horse ❷, insert the syringe into his mouth ❸, and then insert it farther ❹. This syringe is filled with a gastric medication this horse needs to take.

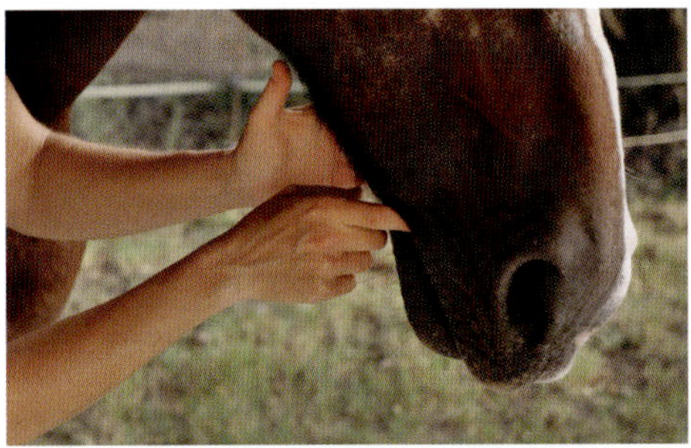

Inserting your finger into the corner of the horse's mouth and then rewarding him can help him accept the syringe better. Your other hand shouldn't be restraining or pushing; it can just rest against the horse's jaw, providing steady contact.

Additional step: If your horse is very reluctant to take the syringe into the corner of his mouth, you can add another step between 5 and 6.

Touch the corner of the horse's mouth with your finger, and then click, lift it away, and reward the horse. Repeat, inserting your finger into the horse's mouth as if positioning a bit, and then click, move it away, and reward the horse. You should be able to move on to step 6 after this. If your horse is still nervous and you have trouble inserting the syringe, try setting your finger at the corner of his mouth, waiting for it to open as he expects you to insert it again, and then inserting the syringe instead, keeping your finger where it is. Practicing the Touching the Gums exercise can also help (see page 85).

Common Mistakes

Forgetting to repeat this training after a medication has successfully been given to the horse. Sometimes, medications taste bad, and the horse picks up a negative association with this process even after all your hard work; you need to replace it with more memories of food rewards.

As I describe in Touching Sensitive Places (see page 74), you can ask the horse to stand still by teaching him to touch the palm of your hand with his nose. While you keep your hand there for him, someone else can administer oral medication. However, making this work means:

- Preparing the horse by practicing with the target you're going to use (see the Touching Sensitive Places exercise);
- Familiarizing the horse with the overall procedure using clicker or approach-retreat techniques.

This method is a great choice for particularly nervous horses.

Learning from Experience

In the case of my pony Victor, who was trained to use the "stop button," having him touch someone's hand also keeps his head steady, which is especially useful. My children help me with his care, and they don't have enough experience to manage Victor if he tries to grab the syringe out of their hands, the way he does with me (if he gets impatient, he'll take the syringe in his teeth, and the medication will spill out of his mouth). Asking him to touch one of their hands keeps his mouth still and closed, which makes it much easier for them to give him his medication. I just have to make sure my kids know that they need to stop the procedure if Victor moves his nose away from that hand.

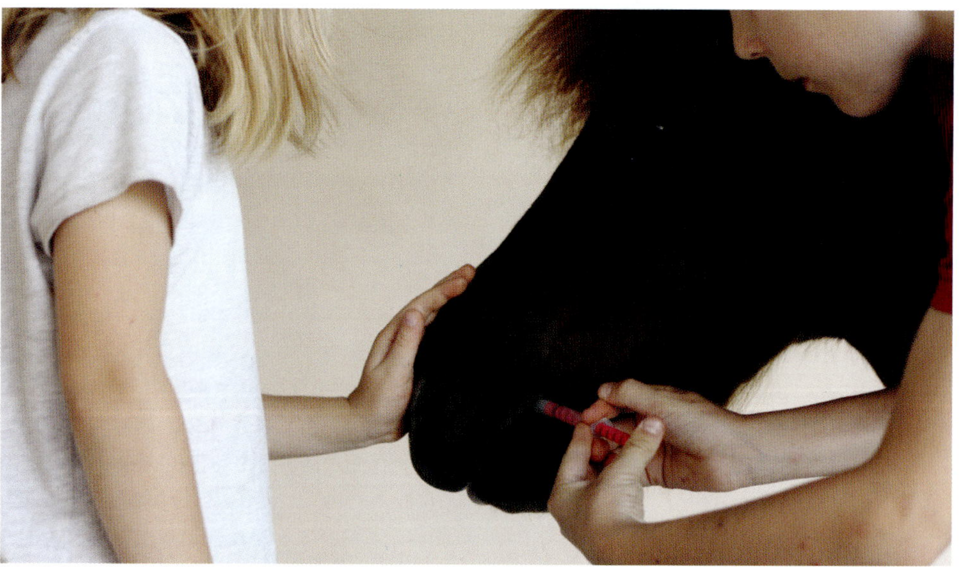

Teaching an equine to use the "stop button" requires us to follow the rules—to stop when the animal asks us to stop—and do it consistently, if we want to keep his trust.

Administering Eye Care

What's the Point?

Your horse might need to allow someone to touch his eye for multiple reasons:

- To rinse it out, if something is in it;
- To treat a condition like uveitis by applying ointment or eye drops;
- To perform an ophthalmologic examination.

Eye conditions (uveitis, ulcers, or keratitis, for example) are very painful for horses. As soon as you notice any discomfort in your horse that's related to his eyes—if one of them doesn't open as far as the other, if either or both are swollen or seeping—contact your veterinarian so they can examine him.

Eye treatments may need to be carried out multiple times a day, as frequently as every 2 hours. Whether you're applying eye drops or ointment, if your horse is constantly moving his head:

- It will be difficult or impossible to apply the medication;

- You'll be in danger;

- Your horse is at risk of injury, especially damage to his cornea, if he moves when you aren't expecting it and the applicator pokes or scrapes the surface of his eye.

Whether you're in an emergency situation already or just hoping to prepare for the possibility in the future, you should handle this exercise the same way. If you feel like it's taking too long, remind yourself that your options are to spend an hour on this the first time through, with a calm animal who understands what he needs to do, or to spend fifteen minutes in a war zone.

If the latter is still tempting, be aware that you're also risking even more problems the next time around—the horse will guess what's coming, and since his defensive reactions last time weren't enough to stop you from messing with his eye, he'll feel like he needs to escalate this time. Of course it's easier to be patient when you're training the horse for future examinations than when your horse's health depends on your ability to provide him with medical care. All the more reason to prepare in advance, whenever you have the option, both for your sake so you know exactly what to do and have

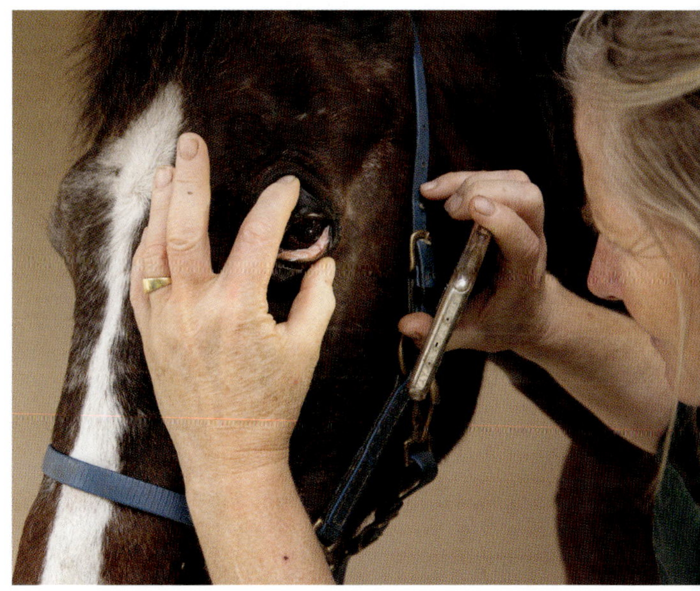

Train your horse to allow his eyes to be examined—here, a light is shining into this horse's eye.

confidence in your ability to request the behavior your need from your horse; and for your horse so he knows he has nothing to fear from the procedure and can trust you.

What You'll Need

- Sterile compresses;
- Vials of saline solution.

What You Want the Horse to Do

- Stay still even when someone is touching his eye (if you use approach-retreat).
- Move his eye toward your hand himself and hold his head still (if you use clicker training).

✦ What You Do

With a horse who's free to move, you can use either approach-retreat (see Touching Sensitive Places, page 74) or voluntary contact (see page 79). I'll explain the voluntary contact technique here, because in my experience, it yields fantastic results and is both rapid and effective. If your horse understands the Touch-Click exercise (see page 47) and knows the rules that govern the arrival of his rewards, this should be a pretty quick process. It'll go even faster if you've already trained your horse in the "stop button" (see Touching Sensitive Places, page 74); you just need to change the area you want him to touch to your hand from his nose to his eye. In 30 minutes, including breaks, you should be able to earn the cooperation of a previously reluctant horse. If you're in a hurry, you can start this exercise immediately, without doing any other exercises—but be careful and take as much time with it as you can, especially if you aren't experienced with these training methods.

✦ Step by Step: Voluntary Contact with a Neutral Area

This exercise involves helping the horse understand that he needs to move toward your hand and keep his head still.

Position yourself at the horse's shoulder and double-check his "politeness": he should be looking straight ahead, and you should be able to click and reward him without him coming around to look for his treat himself. If this training isn't solid yet, you should go through this exercise in "protected contact"—with him on one side of a physical barrier like a stall door, and you on the other side. You should also use this method with a horse who has violent reactions when people try to touch his head.

Once you have the horse standing still and looking straight ahead:

1. Move your hand toward his throatlatch or cheek without actually touching him. He'll probably turn his head; he may think this is a reward coming, and touch you first. This is fine—that's the goal, even if he's not doing it for the right reasons right now!

2. As soon as he touches you, click, and then lower your hand.

 — **PREPARING YOUR HORSE OR DONKEY FOR VETERINARY CARE**

3. Reward him with your other hand. This is especially important if your horse isn't very "polite" and you don't have time to teach or review politeness with him; if you try to reward him with the same hand you're using to touch him, he might smell the traces of treats on your fingers and try to grab your hand.

4. Start again: hold your hand near his face but don't touch him, and wait for him to come to you. If he still hasn't touched your hand himself after 30 seconds, move your hand up or down, just an inch or two. This movement can remind him that he hasn't solved the problem and gotten his reward yet. Once he touches your hand with his face, click, and reward him with your other hand.

If your horse simply isn't interested in your hand at all, during the first three tries—and only the first three—you should be the one to touch him, after 30 seconds of waiting; as soon as you touch him, while you're still touching him, click, and then take your hand away and reward him with the other hand. Then start again, waiting with your hand not touching him. He should make the connection and start moving to touch your hand on his own.

As you continue, make sure your horse is touching your hand, with his cheek or jaw, quickly and steadily: you present him with your hand, and within two seconds or less, he touches it. Achieve this three times

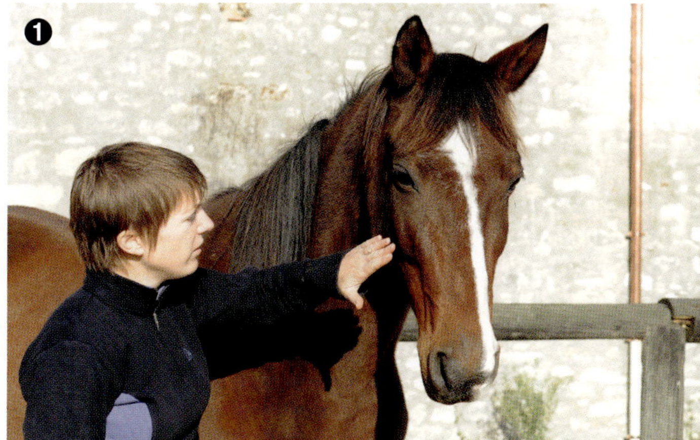

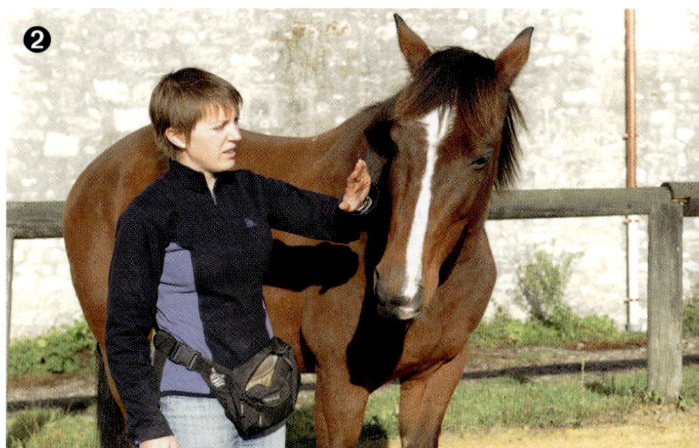

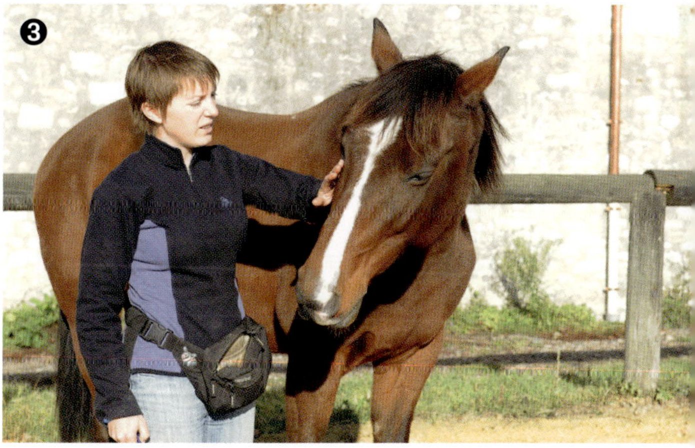

Your hand is the target the horse needs to learn you want him to touch—first with a part of his head other than his nose ❶, and then you can gradually refine the target until he knows he needs to touch your hand with his eye ❷). It should always be the horse who touches you, not you touching him ❸.

in a row, clicking and rewarding him each time, and you're ready to ask him to prolong the contact. Stick with the cheek for the moment so you can keep practicing without asking him to offer a sensitive area like his nostrils or his eyes, which would be harder for him. Your horse is unlikely to have any strong negative associations with being touched on the cheek, so he shouldn't be reluctant to touch it to your hand (unless he has a dental problem that's causing cheek pain). The next time you offer your hand and he touches it with his cheek again, don't click right away:

1. Count to two.

2. Click (it's normal for the horse to move away from your hand at this point).

3. Move your hand away, if you're still touching the horse at all.

4. Reward him with your other hand.

5. Repeat, increasing the duration of the contact before you click.

6. Alternate between longer durations and shorter ones.

Teaching your horse to hold this contact with your hand will mean he keeps his head still later, when you're going to be juggling the eye dropper and a cotton pad and trying to hold his eye open at the same time … In other words, you're teaching him patience!

You can also ask your horse to turn his head slightly toward you, which will keep you safer if he feels the need to strike with a foreleg. To do this, just hold your hand in line with your body instead of out to one side of you; if the horse wants to touch it with his cheek, he's going to have to bend his neck a little more toward you. At first, you won't ask him to hold this contact, just to give you a touch; then, once he's adjusted to the new position, you can increase duration again.

✦ Step by Step: Voluntary Contact with Sensitive Places

You'll now start to change the area you're asking the horse to touch you with. This time, instead of positioning your hand near his cheek, hold it closer to his cheekbone, just under his eye. Follow the same steps as when you were asking him to touch your hand with his cheek. If he understood that part correctly, it'll take him two or three click-reward cycles to understand that you want him to touch you with the area your hand is close to. Increase the duration of the touches, and remember you can ask him to turn his head toward you a little if you keep your hand in line with you instead of off to one side of you.

And then—you guessed it—the next step is to hold your hand near his eye (about 8 inches away).

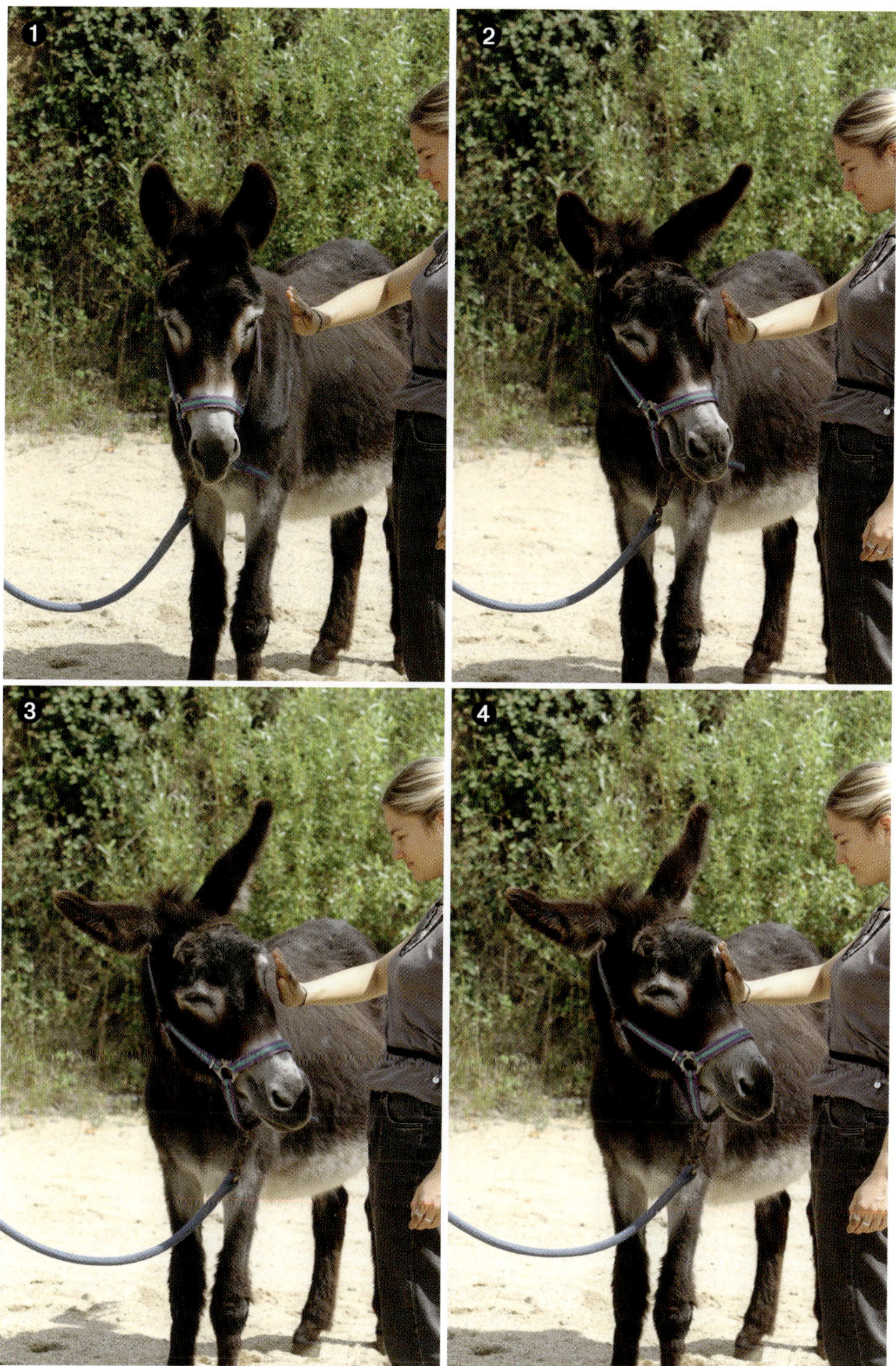

This donkey touches the trainer's hand with his eye; she waits one extra second to click, and then another, and little by little, she increases the duration of the touch.

Some horses will pick up on this principle very quickly, and will move their eye toward your hand immediately. But this is a very sensitive spot, and your horse may offer to touch your hand with his cheekbone again, or his cheek, by raising his head or moving it away. If this happens, hold your hand a little closer to his eye to ask again. If your horse moves toward your hand without raising or lowering his head to change the zone of contact, click immediately and reward him with your other hand, even if he hasn't touched you yet. Just make sure you don't do the touching! If he's the one who's deciding to touch you every time, you'll be able to provide care to him without needing any restraints at all.

If you're in an emergency situation and you can't put off care for long, at this stage—as long as the horse isn't upset—you can:

1. Hold him by the noseband of his halter (see Grasping the Halter Firmly on page 59).

2. Touch his eye gently.

3. Click immediately.

4. Move your hand away and release his halter.

5. Reward him.

Work through the stages of contact with the eye the same way you did for the cheek and the cheekbone.

With Both Hands Busy

This step shouldn't be done until your horse is good at the preceding steps. Progress with this method can be surprisingly fast (within 30 minutes, breaks included), but you shouldn't rush through it; don't hesitate to end the session and continue another day, as long as you're concluding on a good note. Once your horse is willing to touch your hand with his eye, you'll simulate treatment:

- Hold the horse's eyelids apart with one hand.
- Apply eye drops or ointment with the other hand, being very careful not to touch the surface of the eye with the applicator.

Both of your hands will be occupied, so you won't be able to use a clicker. You can still mark good behavior with a noise like a click of your tongue (not the same click you use to ask the horse to walk or trot). You can teach the horse the meaning of this noise in just a couple of click-reward cycles. Ask him for something he already does well (the Statue exercise, or one of the earlier, easier steps in this exercise), and when he does it, wait one second and:

- Click your tongue.
- Click with the clicker.
- Reward him.

Repeat a few times, and then watch his reaction as you click only your tongue and then reward him. If he's started to respond the same way to the click of your tongue as he did to the sound of the clicker, you're all set: he's made the connection. If he doesn't seem to get it, repeat, asking for a behavior and marking it with both kinds of clicks and then rewarding him, and then try using your tongue alone again.

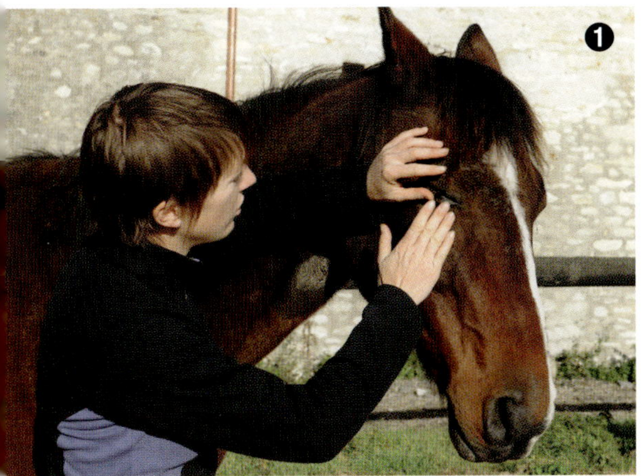

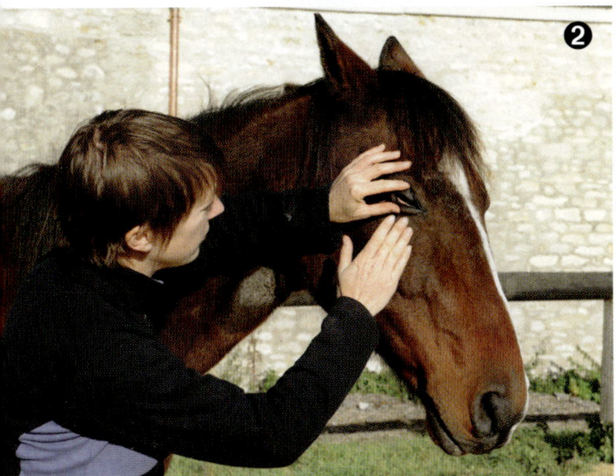

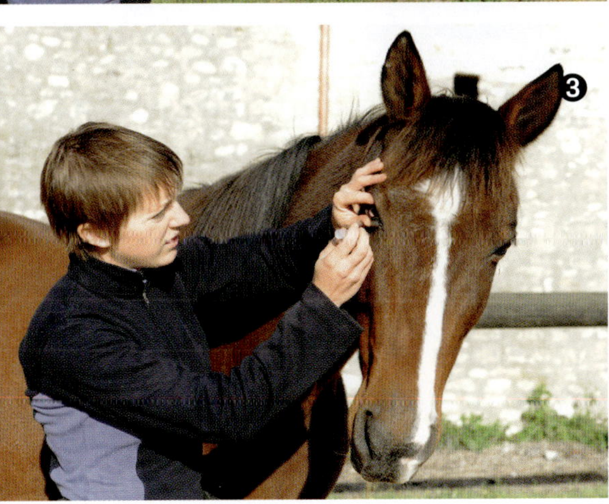

This training will start to resemble treatment of the eye with both hands ❶, and then treatment involving more intrusive manipulation of the eyelids ❷, and then, last but not least, bringing an applicator close to the eye ❸.

More Intrusive Treatment

The next piece of the training puzzle is for the horse to accept you touching and manipulating his eyelids. You probably haven't done this before. Wash your hands before you start!

1. Ask your horse to touch your hand with his eye for a few seconds.

2. Move your fingers over his eyelids.

3. If the horse stays still, click your tongue.

4. Lift your hand away.

5. Reward him.

Little by little, work your way gradually to the point where you can use your thumb against the lower eyelid and the index finger of the same hand against the upper eyelid to open your horse's eye wider. Don't hesitate to ask your vet to show you how.

Each time the horse cooperates, give him a click with your tongue to let him know that was the right thing to do, and then reward him. Switch back to just asking him to touch your hand with his eye a few times, and always end a session asking him for an easier step than the one you were working on during the session. Don't get greedy!

Involving the Other Hand

The next new element to introduce here is your other hand approaching the eye, with the horse maintaining contact and your "original" hand holding the horse's eyelids open. At first, just moving your other hand toward the eye should result in a click and a reward if the horse stands still without moving away; then bring your hand closer, until you're touching the corner of the horse's eye with it.

Then follow the same steps while holding a closed bottle of saline eye solution in your hand. This seemingly minor change can cause the horse to withdraw sharply—if he's had bad experiences with eye care in the past, there's a big difference between your empty hand and your hand with that bottle in it, for him.

Work your way up to applying a few drops of saline to the inner corner of the horse's eye.

The last step in this part of the exercise is to squirt a little bit of saline solution into the eye itself. This can surprise a horse no matter how carefully you do it, so even if the horse raises his head abruptly in response, click and reward him, and then go back to a simpler step so you can end on a good note.

Practicing these steps will make it much easier for you to care for your horse's eyes; even if he's in considerable pain, he'll recognize a familiar routine and do his best to cooperate. This was actually proven directly by a study[65] following the same procedure I've described in this exercise.

If you have to provide care to an untrained horse in an emergency, you can speed up by starting with the section "Step by Step: Voluntary

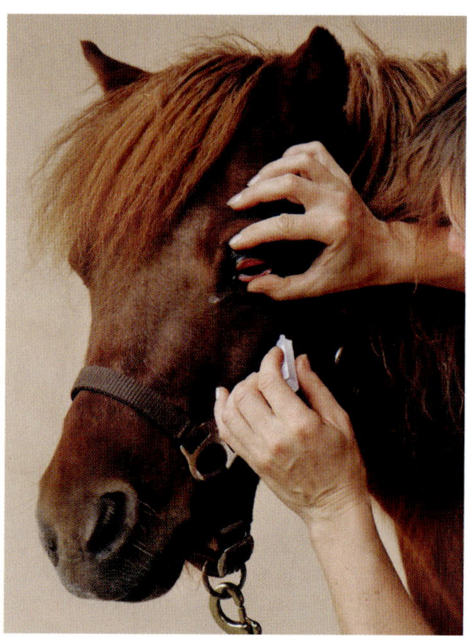

Even working without a helper, and with both of your hands occupied, you'll be able to apply treatment to your horse's eyes with precision.

Learning from Experience

If your horse should end up with something stuck in his eye—piercing his eyeball—you shouldn't ask for contact with the eye itself, but rather with the area just below it, using the tips of your fingers. This will make it easier for the vet to remove the object; the horse will be holding his head still. I once had to remove a splinter from a pony's eye myself, because my vet couldn't come right away. I asked someone to help me by rewarding him whenever I clicked my tongue, and I removed the splinter—which was almost an inch long—from the pony's eyeball with a pair of tweezers. I treated the wound with medication prescribed by the vet, and the pony didn't suffer any aftereffects. All the training I'd done in advance helped a lot!

Contact with Sensitive Places" (see page 74), applying light restraint to the horse's halter.

1. Follow the same steps, up to and including "Involving the Other Hand."

2. Take a break and leave the horse alone for a few minutes.

3. Ask someone else for help, either to hold the halter and then release it whenever you click, or to apply medication or treatment to the eye.

4. Have the halter held at the noseband, and then click, release the restraint, and reward the horse (resuming with a very simple exercise).

5. Open the eyelids of the eye you need to treat (this step must be done by whoever is going to treat the eye, not by the person holding the halter); click, stop, and reward the horse.

6. Repeat, applying the medication this time, and then click, move your hands away from the horse's eye, and reward him.

7. Finish with another simple exercise the horse can do easily, and click and reward him again.

If you or whoever is applying medication cannot get it into the eye on the first try, you still need to click, stop, and reward the horse; he did his job, and he shouldn't be deprived of a reward for cooperating well. Little by little, you should start to feel able to do this alone, and to forgo even the restraint of the halter eventually; the horse will perceive this easing of pressure over time.[66] If you want to watch a video of a pony cooperating with treatment for uveitis, check the references at the end of this book.

Troubleshooting

"My horse moves his head while he's touching my hand."

When you ask for continuous contact, your horse is turning his head slightly to the other side, or

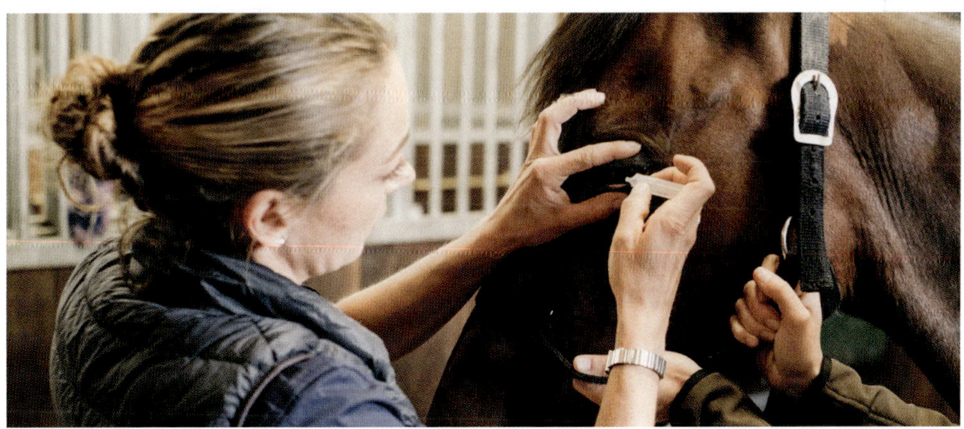

In an emergency, restraining the horse's head for a few seconds, releasing it, and then clicking and giving him a food reward can help him understand that he should hold his head still, even if he's in pain.

raising or lowering his head, making it harder for you to provide care. If this happens, when he starts to move, take your hand away; position it in a new place where his head will have to be in a better position in order for him to touch it, and wait for him to come to it and touch it again. Click, take your hand away, and reward him. Start again, and keep asking him to hold this new and improved position for a longer duration.

Common Mistakes

- Moving to create contact; you have to leave it up to the horse to close the distance between his face and your hand.
- Keeping your hand close to the horse's eye after clicking, instead of moving it away.

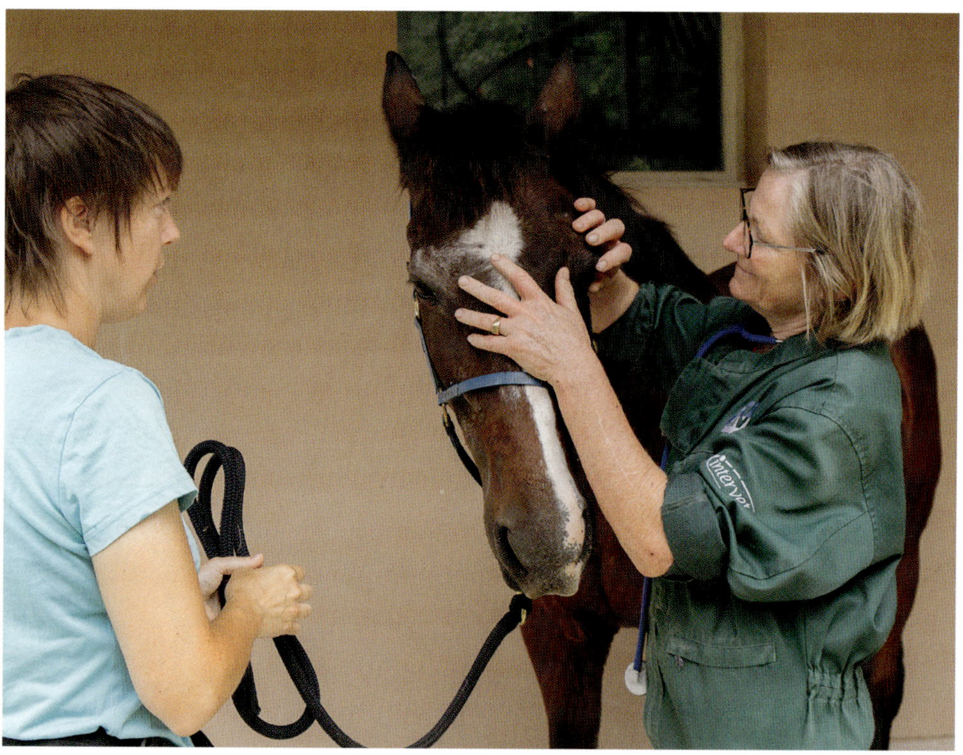

Having another person manipulate the horse's eyes is a whole new step to add on to this exercise. Don't be surprised if he has trouble with it, even if he was cooperating with you really well. Reward him for even very short spans of cooperation with a new person.

Positioning a Limb

What's the Point?

Being able to direct a horse's foot onto a support is essential if your veterinarian wants to take an x-ray to diagnose damage to the musculo-skeletal system (in a case of lameness, for example). Usually, even if a horse will lift his leg, he won't put it down in the right spot; you'll have to pick it up again and reposition it, and then he won't wait long enough to let the x-ray machine finish, and you'll have to start over from the top.

What You'll Need

- Some wooden blocks an inch thick, wide enough across for a horse to place his foot on the surface with room to spare and strong enough to support his weight on that leg.
- A car mat (preferably a rubber one, for easy cleaning).

What You Want the Horse to Do

- Step on a block when you ask him to.
- Bend his leg a little bit but stand still.

✦ What You Do

You can just pick up the horse's leg and put his foot wherever you want. The issue is that the horse will probably move it again, if he isn't comfortable with its position thanks to the change in the distribution of his weight and his balance, and the quality of any diagnostic image will suffer for it. Focus on teaching the horse to understand that you're asking for something specific that won't last forever, and he'll do a better job standing still despite having his leg in an unusual position. Clicker training is precise and effective for this exercise.

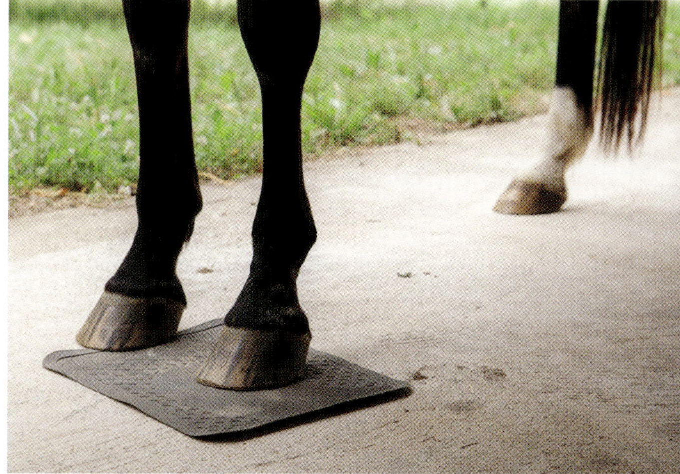

Placing the horse's foot is one thing. Getting him to hold that foot still on a specific surface is another. Fortunately, this is yet another behavior you can train your horse to offer when you ask for it.

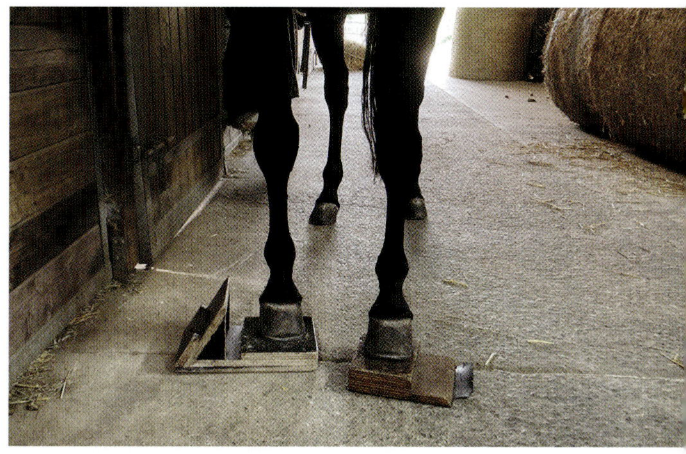

Blocks are necessary in order to x-ray a horse's foot. Training your horse to place his feet on a small surface that's made of a different material from the rest of the footing around him will make diagnostic imaging of his feet and legs much easier.

You'll need a helper to do this exercise. It can be done as preparation on the day the vet is going to come even if you haven't practiced it before then, although it will work better if you've already practiced asking the horse to hold still with the Statue exercise (see page 38).

Stepping on a Block

1. Ask the horse to lift his foot, and position it on a block; as soon as it touches down fully, click, lift it away and let him set it down somewhere else, and reward him.

2. Place the foot back on the block, and if the horse tries to shift his weight to it, click, lift it away and let him set it down somewhere else, and reward him.

3. If the horse doesn't shift his weight onto the foot you've moved, ask a helper to lean on his opposite shoulder, or to pull on his tail if you're working with a hind foot—the moment the horse begins to put weight onto the foot you've moved, click, release his foot, and reward him.

4. Once the horse is putting weight on the foot willingly, wait for one second, click, and reward him; keep going if the horse is willing to stay in position. The vet should now be able to take an x-ray. If the horse still isn't in a stable stance, ask him for a shorter duration, let him take his foot off the block, and then work on extending the duration again.

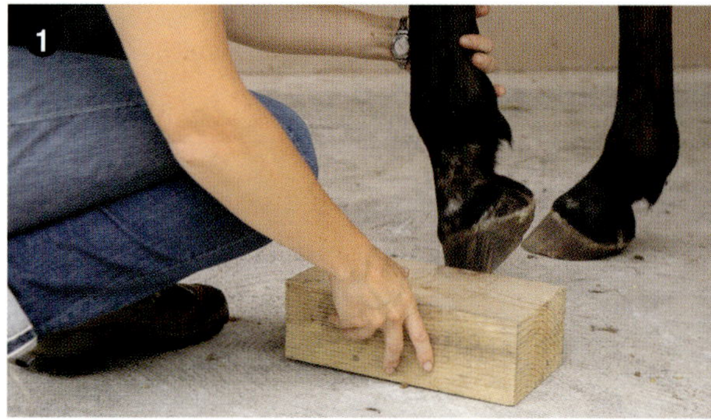

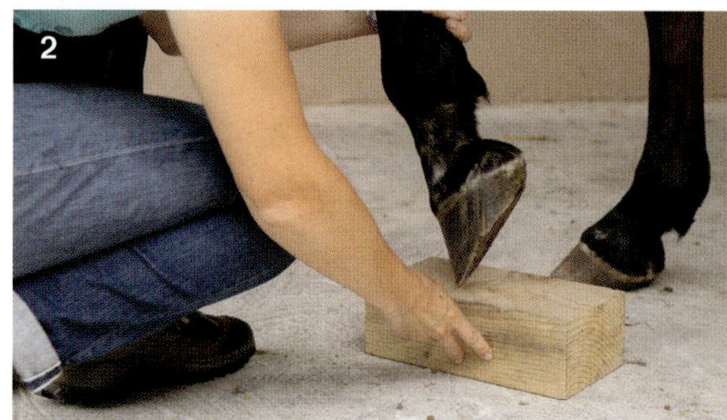

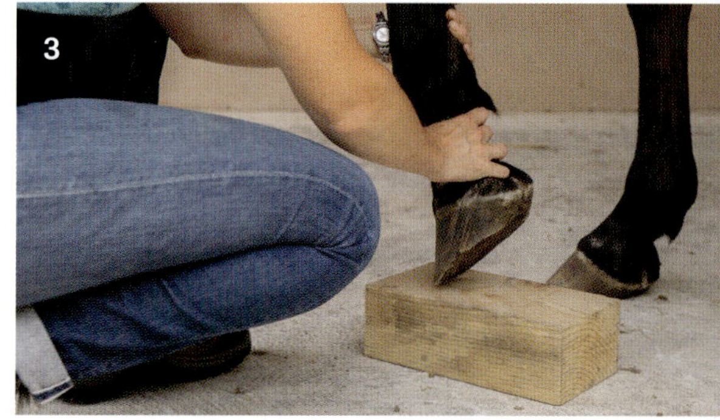

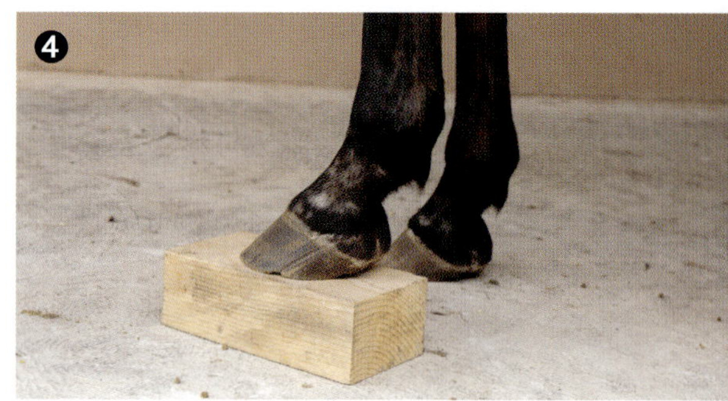

These photos show the steps of moving the horse's foot onto a block. Each step should earn a click and a reward for the horse before you try to chain them together.

Positioning a Limb Without Support

1. Move the limb into the position you want.

2. Hold the limb in place and click; someone other than the person handling the leg should reward the horse.

3. Click and reward at intervals during the procedure (over 30 times, for a duration of one minute).

Common Mistakes

- Letting go of the leg completely if the horse lifts his foot instead of setting it down.
- Pulling or forcing the horse's leg into place, in an effort to avoid the first mistake! Hold onto the leg, but follow the movement the horse is making instead of fighting it, and wait until the horse has stopped trying to move before returning the limb to the position you want.

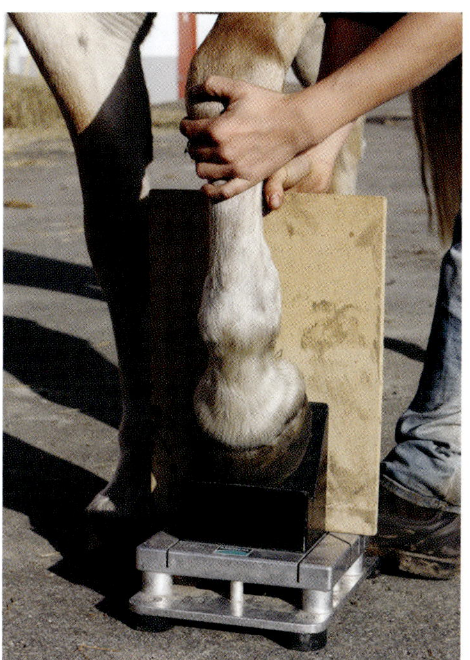

Some x-rays require the hoof to be suspended without any weight resting on it. Here, this board is simulating the angle of an x-ray plate.

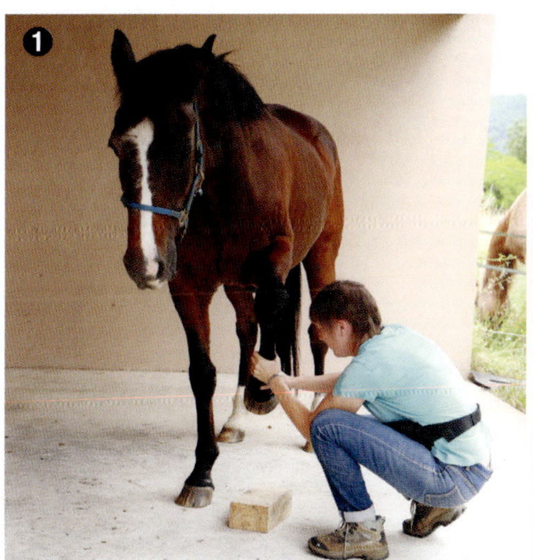

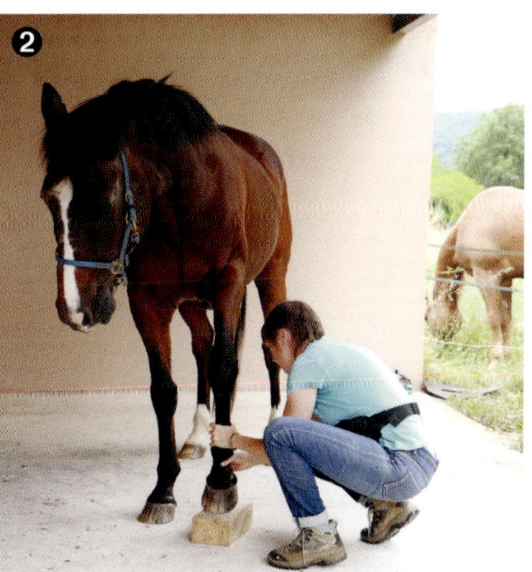

If the horse tries to pull his leg away, follow his movement without letting go of his leg ❶—don't try to fight it. It will come down better when you move it back into position if you aren't forcing it ❷. And don't forget to click, reward the horse, and take breaks.

Weighing with a Scale

What's the Point?

Knowing a horse's weight is crucial in order to administer medication in the right dosage (dewormers, antibiotics) and monitor his body condition, which can be an indicator of health or growth. It's possible to estimate a horse's weight using barymetric formulas based on the horse's size, chest circumference, and breed (the formula for a draft horse's weight isn't the same as the formula for a saddle horse's). But having more precise information to work with is better, especially if surgery is necessary. Equine veterinary clinics usually have scales for this purpose—but the change in surface footing can worry horses to the point where they refuse to stand still on it, or won't step on it in the first place. You probably won't have a scale like this at home, but you can still train your horse to cooperate when you ask him to put his feet on an unfamiliar surface, which will make your life, your vet's life, and any veterinary assistants' lives easier. It will also help make it easier for you to get your horse into a truck or a trailer.

What You Want the Horse to Do

Place his feet on an unfamiliar surface, and then stand still.

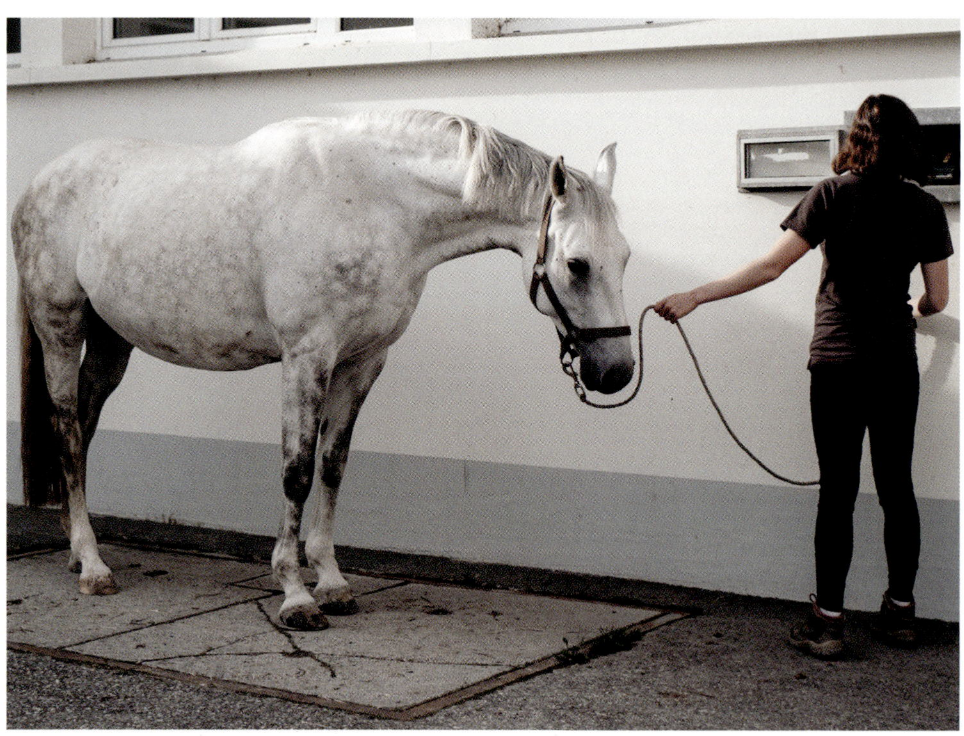

You can practice having your horse hold still, which will serve you well in this exercise.

PREPARING YOUR HORSE OR DONKEY FOR VETERINARY CARE

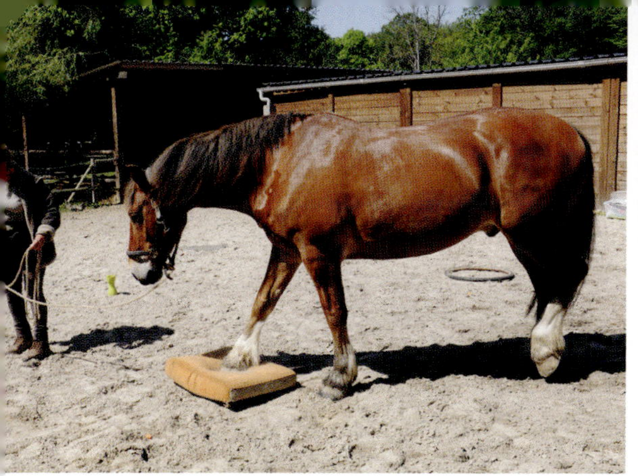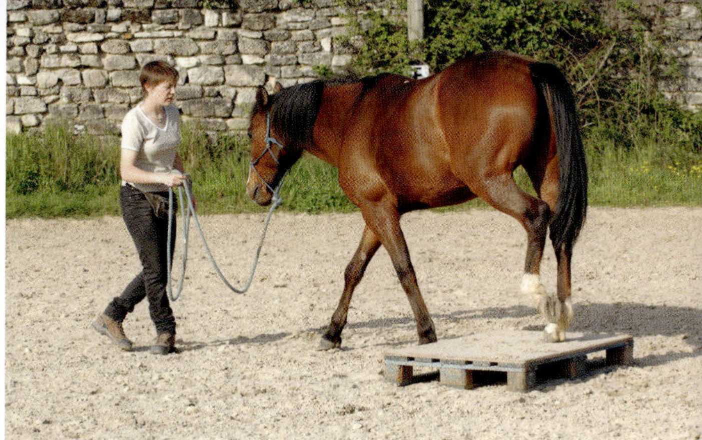

Train your horse to step onto different surfaces, and then to stand still on them. In the photo on the left, the unfamiliar surface is a sofa cushion; on the right, a reinforced pallet.

What You'll Need

You only need one item from the list below to get started, but the more surfaces you can teach your horse to accept, the better off he'll be. Some of these options are more expensive than others; skip anything that isn't in your budget. They're also a variety of different materials, so they'll make different kinds of noises and react differently to the horse's weight (cushions and mattresses will compress, wood won't)—these are opportunities to surprise your horse, if he's the type who always already knows how to do everything!

- Rubber car mats, scraps of carpeting or linoleum.
- Plastic tarpaulins.
- Old sofa cushions, old foam mattresses.
- Wooden construction pallets, reinforced with extra boards.
- A podium (this has to be solid and able to hold the weight of a horse, so skip it if you aren't sure whether you can find one that will hold up).

✦ What You Do

For both parts of this exercise (stepping onto a new surface and then staying there), you can work alone, with the horse in a halter, in an area open enough that the horse can move around the surface you're offering him so he doesn't feel like he has to jump over it if he doesn't want to walk on it. Whether you should be at the horse's shoulder or facing him depends on the situation. Don't crouch down if he's putting a foot on the surface, and don't let yourself get trapped in a corner or a tight space, or you might get jostled. If your horse gets scared—by the noise his foot makes when he sets it on a plastic tarpaulin, for example— he might jump over it, and you need to be able to stay out of his way. You should also avoid working around protruding objects and sharp or solid edges (jump standards, buckets, chairs, and so on) that could hurt or trip you or your horse, or that could tangle up your horse's lead rope.

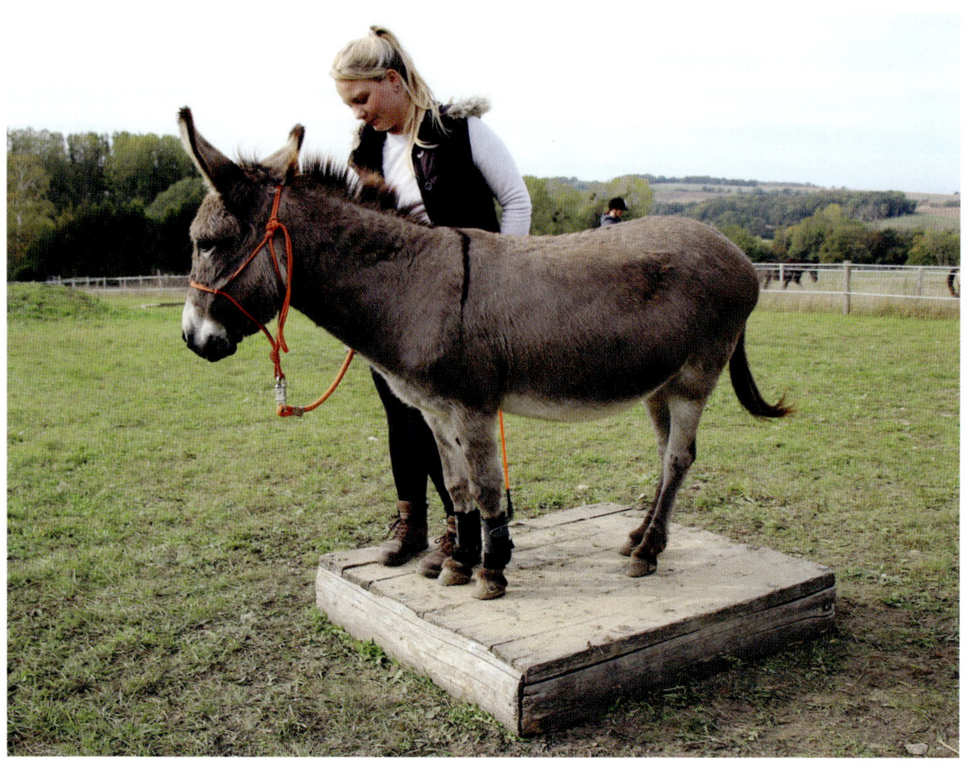

Crossing surfaces in-hand in unusual locations builds this donkey's confidence; he'll have a much easier time positioning himself on a vet's scale or getting into a trailer after this.

I recommend positioning yourself at the horse's shoulder when he's crossing a tarpaulin; the sound of plastic surprises most horses, and they'll speed up or even jump. If you're positioned at the shoulder, with a lead rope that's at least 12 feet long, you should be at a safe distance but you won't lose hold of the lead rope. When it comes to tarpaulins, this position also gives you an advantage in that you can familiarize the horse with the sound it makes when *you* walk on it.

For other kinds of surfaces, though, I think facing the horse is fine. The horse can perceive your attention on him through the direction of your body and your gaze, because he's sensitive to both,[69] and that encourages him to interact with you, and to look for solutions to the problems you're presenting to him.

✦ Step by Step: Pressure and Release

You'll apply pressure to the horse's halter with the lead rope, and then release that pressure as soon as the horse responds to it (by moving forward, lowering his head to examine the surface, or placing his foot on the surface). This is the principle of negative reinforcement.

 — PREPARING YOUR HORSE OR DONKEY FOR VETERINARY CARE

1. Guide the horse toward the surface.

2. Let him lower his head to sniff it and inspect it.

3. Ask him to take a step.

4. Ask him to put one front foot on the surface.

5. Ask him to put both front feet on the surface.

6. Ask him to put a hind foot on the surface also.

7. Ask him to put all four feet on the surface.

8. Ask him to stand still on the surface.

Common Mistakes

- Releasing the pressure on the lead rope when the horse moves backward or away from the surface; follow the movement and maintain pressure instead.
- Putting too much pressure on the horse when he needs time to examine the surface; let him lower his head and touch the surface with his nose, and wait until he's done before you ask for anything else.

✦ Step by Step: With the Clicker

1. Guide your horse as close as he's willing to get to the surface. If he shows signs of worry as you ask him to come closer, then your first session is going to be about letting him adjust to the presence of this surface or object. If he looks at it, click and reward him.

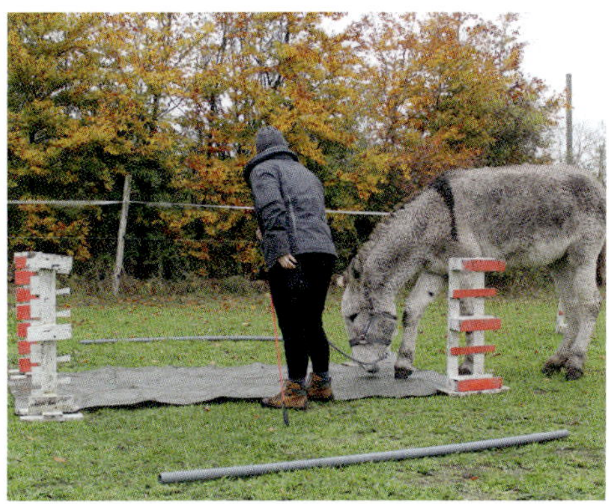

Step 2: It's important to let the animal inspect the unfamiliar surface closely without putting pressure on the lead rope.

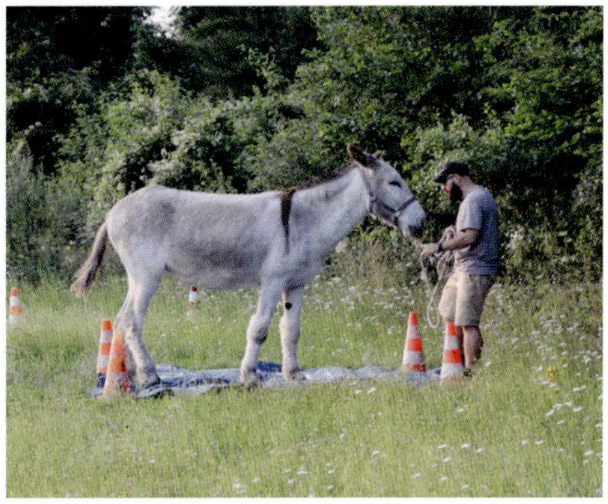

Step 7: Asking the equine to bring his other hind foot onto the tarpaulin.

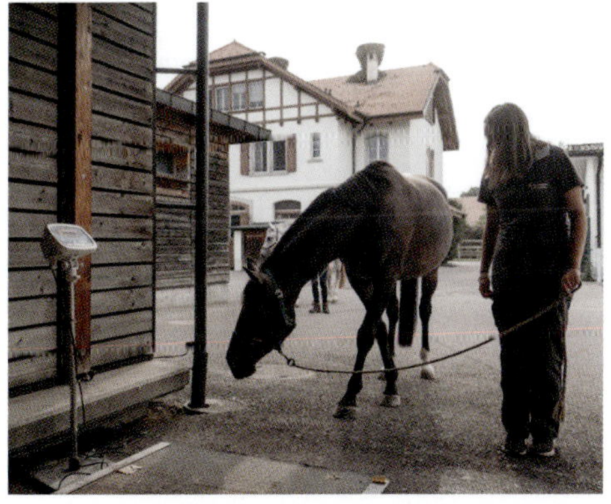

The mare is guided as close as she's willing to get to the scale, and then allowed to sniff them and touch them. You might be able to tell from the photo that she's snorting a little, which is a sign of worry. This scale is designed with a step up, which is an extra obstacle.

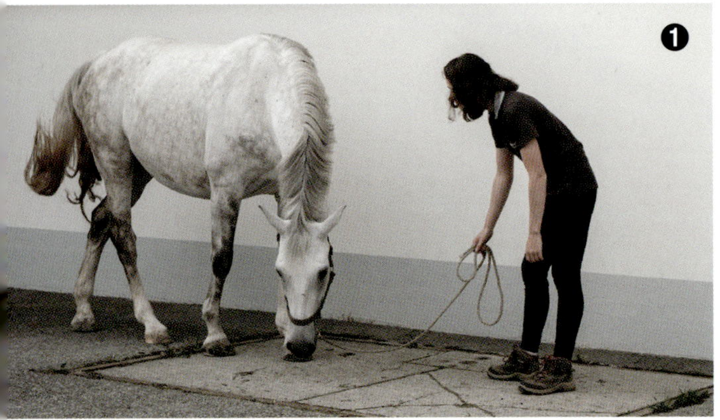 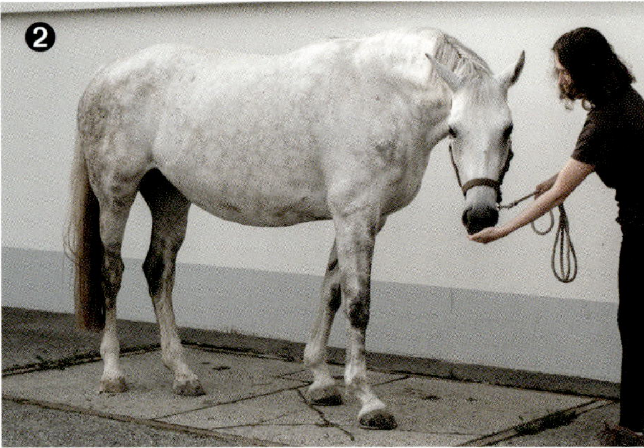

The horse lowers his head and walks onto the unfamiliar surface on his own ❶; his cooperation and willingness to explore will be rewarded ❷.

2. It shouldn't take long for your horse to lower his head to sniff, touch, and get a better look at the surface. Click when he does this, and reward him. If he paws at it or puts a foot on it on his own (sometimes without having smelled it first), that's great—click and reward him. Walking across the surface to give him the reward can reassure him and encourage him to do the same.

3. If you didn't do it during the previous step, now's the time to walk across the surface yourself to demonstrate for the horse the noise it makes; click and reward him if he pays attention, or, better yet, if he stands still while you walk.

Common Mistakes

- Clicking when the horse steps on the surface—I know, it doesn't sound like a mistake! But it's better to click when your horse starts to lift his leg back up, so you don't end up teaching him to paw at the surface.

- Letting him stay on the surface when he's only halfway on it. As soon as his front feet are planted, keep moving him forward, or else he might start pawing.

- Progressing through both front legs and both hind legs in one session. Focus on the front legs during the first few sessions, and leave it at that.

If your horse doesn't try to set a foot on the surface, then use the clicker and a target:

- Encourage him to move toward you by offering him a target to touch with his nose (see page 47)—make sure he can reach it without having to step on the surface.

- Put the target a little farther away, so he has to set one foot on the surface to get to it, or even just the toe of one foot.

- Click and reward every bit of progress.

Your horse will start to understand what you want from him very quickly, and will deliberately put a foot on the surface. Click and reward him for this, and feel free to stop and return to this exercise in another session.

If your horse doesn't try to put a foot on the surface, use a combination of pressure and the clicker:

- Apply light pressure to the lead rope.
- Click and release the pressure at the same time, as soon as your horse starts to move in the right direction (shifting his weight forward, moving his head forward, or moving a hind foot forward, even if his front legs aren't moving yet).
- Give him a reward.

Combining negative reinforcement (the pressure on the lead rope) and positive reinforcement (the reward), follow the same steps as on the previous page with the target technique. Little by little, your horse will position his front legs on the surface, and then his hind legs (if the size of the surface allows for it) you need to:

- Ask the horse to stand still with one or both front feet on the surface.
- Vary the material—bring in another unfamiliar surface.

Don't position yourself as you would for the Statue exercise, or the horse might not know whether he's supposed to step forward or stand still.

✦ Troubleshooting

"My horse goes around the surface and comes toward me."

In this situation, you might not have encouraged his interest in investigating the surface enough; sniffs, or even glances toward the surface if he's stopped wanting to sniff, need to be clicked for and rewarded. If he goes around the surface, reposition yourself so you're facing it with him on the other side of it. If he isn't facing you and turns a little bit, that's okay. If you keep encouraging his interest in the surface, he'll start trying to cross it.

"He didn't see the surface and stepped over it without stepping on it."

If he stepped over the surface without touching it at all, then it's quite possible that he *did* see it and knows exactly where it is—and exactly where he's putting his feet in order to avoid it. You can try using a larger surface, something the horse can't step over. Reposition yourself so the horse is on one side and you're on the other. Another tip: start with a folded sheet or tarpaulin, and then gradually increase the width of the exposed surface by unfolding it little by little.[70]

"He went across the surface in one direction, but he won't cross back over it, so now he won't go over it at all."

Objective number 1 is to get the horse's feet onto the surface; objective number 2 could be to go in one direction, and then the other, but it doesn't have to be. Have the horse cross in one direction once he's put his feet on the surface, and leave it at that; you can work on crossing in the other direction another time, once the horse is really comfortable going one way. Remember, you should focus on one stage at a time.

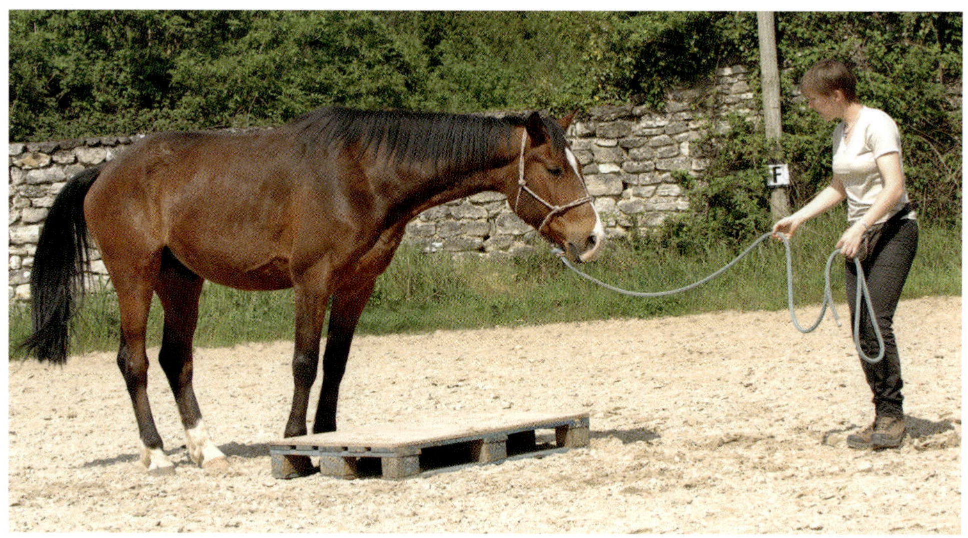

Progress isn't always linear! If the horse isn't comfortable, he might make a first attempt, but then refuse to try again. Work in small steps and short sessions, and go back to a previous step whenever you need to.

"My horse stepped on the surface once, but he won't do it again."

It's possible that your timing was off, and you clicked too late, when the horse had already moved his foot back off the surface. These things happen. If he tried it once, eventually he'll be willing to try it again. Don't hesitate to encourage him by going back to a previous step, namely clicking and rewarding him for sniffing the surface and touching it with his nose. Another possibility is that setting his foot down scared him, if the surface made a noise he wasn't expecting (crunching with a plastic tarpaulin, the hollow noise of a wooden pallet). You can help him get used to it by making the same noise yourself, and clicking and rewarding him for standing still next to the surface while you're doing it. Alternate between this step and asking him to touch the surface, and eventually he should offer to put a foot on it again. The problem might also be the sensation of touching the surface, if he slipped a little on a wet piece of wood or the object moved when he began to put weight on it (a pallet tipping, a foam mattress compressing). If this is the issue, the solution isn't always straightforward. If the horse isn't too badly frightened, he'll probably try to step on the surface again on his own sooner or later, if you rewarded him amply the first time he did it. If he *is* afraid, he won't want to put his foot on it again, at least not anytime soon. Click and reward him for success with any previous steps he does undertake (sniffing the surface, touching it with his nose, lifting a foreleg even if he doesn't actually set his foot down on the surface).

 — PREPARING YOUR HORSE OR DONKEY FOR VETERINARY CARE

You can also try changing the surface, choosing a new material that won't cause the same problem. Once this exercise is successful with another surface (a sheet, a rubber mat), try with others that also won't tip or deform in response to the horse's weight. Your horse will regain his confidence and his willingness to try to do what you ask him, and later on, you'll be able to ask him to repeat the exercise that scared him.

Teach the Horse a New Signal

Once the horse is willing to set his foot on a new surface, you can teach him a signal for this action, so he'll only put his feet on an object, or stand on it, when you ask him to. Choose a word or a gesture (pointing with your finger, for example).

- Say the word or perform the gesture, just before the horse does the action.
- Click and reward him.
- Repeat this several times in a row (at least two or three times).
- Move a little farther away from the surface, and ask for the Statue for a few seconds.
- Click and reward.
- Give your signal and walk toward the surface—click and reward the horse if he does what you intended him to do.
- Repeat this several times, at a distance that gives the horse a chance to stand still and not anticipate your request before you make it.
- Come closer to the surface, and alternate between the Statue and your signal to step on the surface.

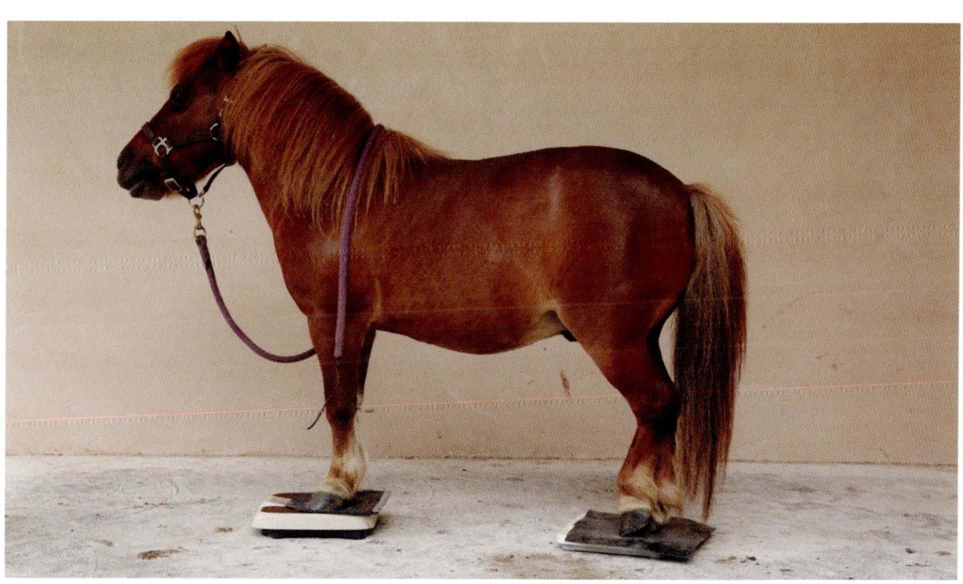

You can weigh equines that are at or under about 450 pounds with two normal scales! Just add the numbers from the scales together. This is a useful trick to help the veterinarian adjust medication dosages for relatively small equines.

Guiding a Horse into a Treatment Room (or Any Location Set Aside for Care)

What's the Point?

In many stables, there's an area set aside for veterinary care. Usually this is the hose-down area. You might not have a space like this at home. Still, think about what you do when your vet arrives for a checkup. Is there anywhere on your property he usually asks you to take your horse, pony, or donkey? If your equine only goes to that location to have unpleasant experiences, he may have negative associations with it. So take him there to do something he'll enjoy!

What You Want the Horse to Do

- Enjoy his time at the location.
- Explore the location freely.

◆ What You Do

The point of this exercise isn't to work on any particular behavior; it's just to give your horse a pleasant experience in a place where he usually has unpleasant experiences. In all of the other exercises, you've made an effort to give your horse positive associations—you'll be doing the same thing here. You can choose to do whatever you think your horse might like: clicker exercises he's already good at (guaranteed food rewards!), feeding him, grooming him (if he likes being groomed) … There are plenty of clicker exercises in this book you can practice, starting with the Statue and Touch-Click. Do them in this veterinary care location.

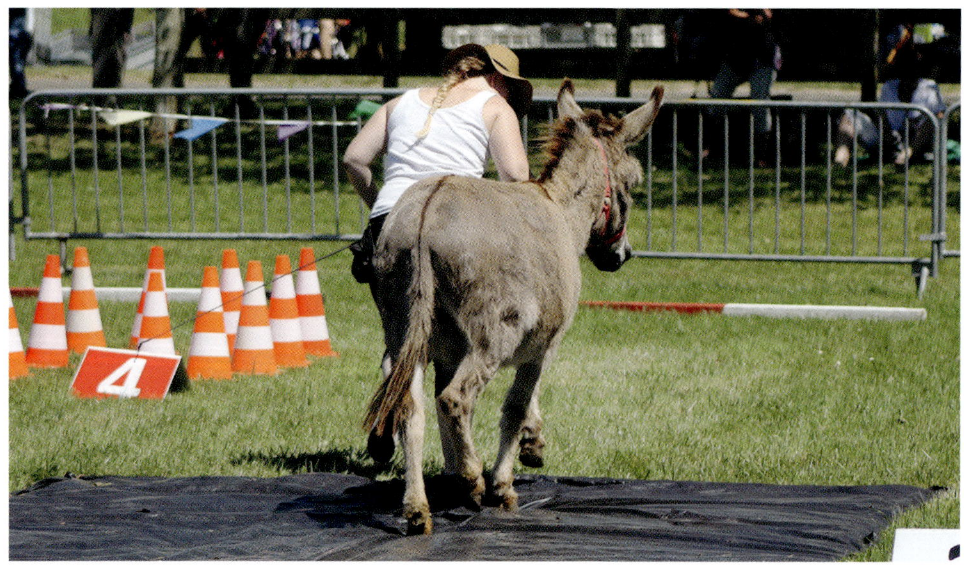

Visiting unfamiliar places such as competition venues prepares you for the day your equine might need to take a trip to a veterinary clinic he's never been to before.

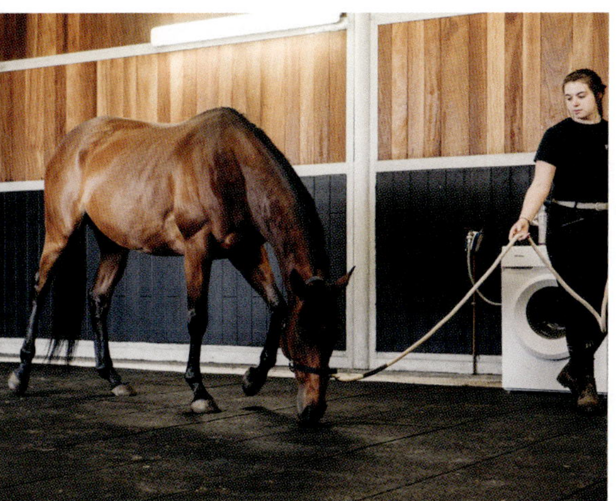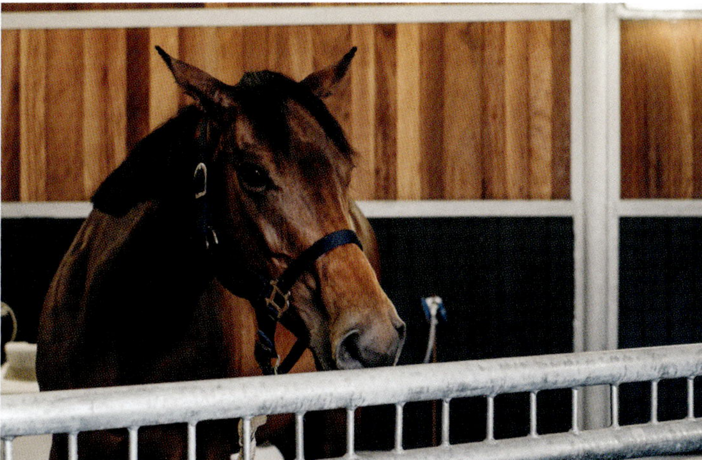

Letting the horse sniff the ground and inspect his surroundings reassures him (left). Allowing him to smell things at his head height is also a good idea (right).

Common Mistakes

- Carrying out nothing but invasive, uncomfortable, painful procedures in the location you've set aside for veterinary care, which means in your horse's mind it's a torture chamber … If you were given flowers or chocolates every time you went to the dentist, and sometimes you didn't even have to get your teeth cleaned, you'd be a lot more relaxed when you *did* get your teeth cleaned—or even if you needed a cavity filled. It's the same for your horse!

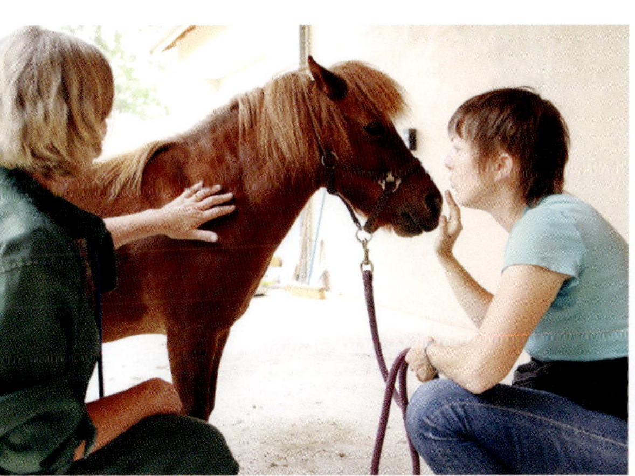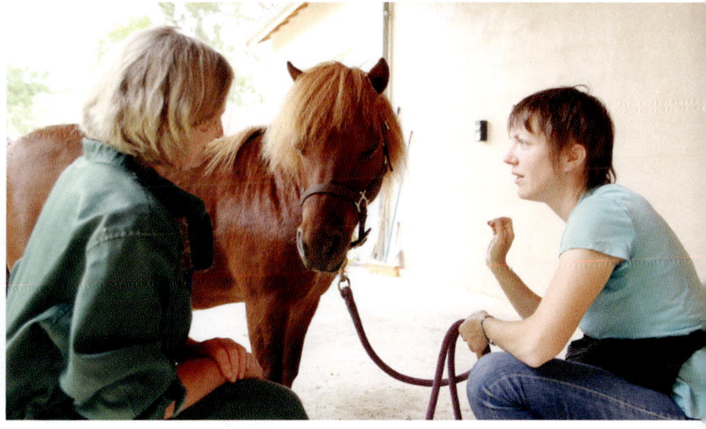

Allowing the equine to look at the person handling him also helps reassure him (left). This pony takes a look and then blinks (right), which is a sign that he's relaxing.

Collecting Urine Samples

What's the Point?

Urine sample analysis is common in some kinds of competitive horse sport, especially those that require doping tests. However, urine samples are also sometimes part of a veterinary examination, because they may help a vet identify or monitor:

- Urinary infections.
- Metabolic issues (myopathy, for example).
- The progression of a pregnancy.

Collection of urine samples is usually done with a container held in the hand or at the end of a handle, to take a sample when a horse is urinating naturally. A urinary catheter is also possible, but less common.

What You'll Need

- A collection container with a handle.

What You Want the Horse to Do

Urinate calmly, next to someone who's extending an object toward a sensitive place.

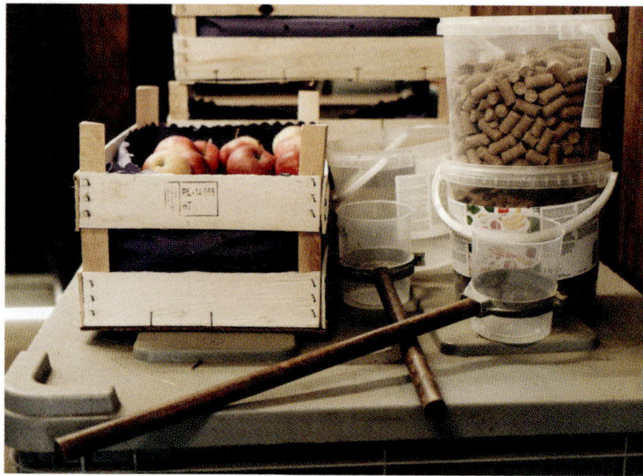

Equipment for collecting a urine sample. Rewards will motivate the horse to cooperate with the procedure.

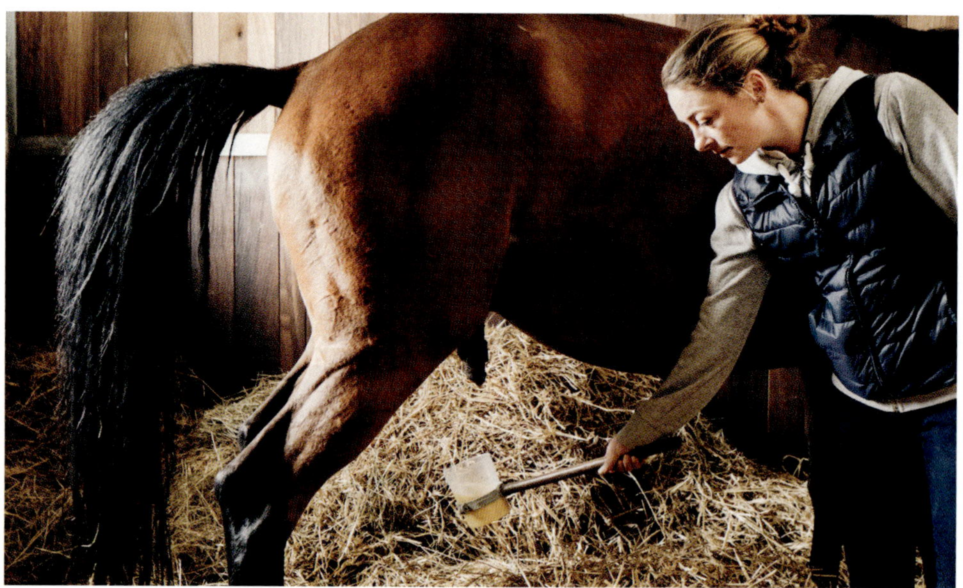

Urine analysis is used in doping tests, but it also helps veterinarians monitor an animal's health.

 — **PREPARING YOUR HORSE OR DONKEY FOR VETERINARY CARE**

✦ What You Do

Usually, horses urinate after exercise, when they're returned to the stable, especially if they have clean bedding to do it into. Sometimes the gap between the horse's daily work and urination can be pretty long! Some horses are also nervous about the container moving around under their bellies, especially male horses, and they may hold back because of it. A horse who's confident and comfortable being touched everywhere (see Touching Sensitive Places on page 74) will be more relaxed, and is more likely to urinate while you're there. Positive reinforcement and precise work with a clicker can help the horse understand what you'd like him to do here.

Begin in a calm setting, and one where the horse is likely to be comfortable urinating: somewhere with absorbent footing (straw, shavings, leaves, or tall grass). Horses usually hate feeling splashing when they urinate! If you've noticed any particular habits governing when your horse urinates, whether he often does it in a specific place or at a specific time, take advantage of it for this exercise.

✦ Step by Step: Approach-Retreat and the Clicker

Your horse should already be trained in the exercises I categorize under "politeness"—see page 34 and following—so you can move around the horse with treats without him bothering you, otherwise, he might start

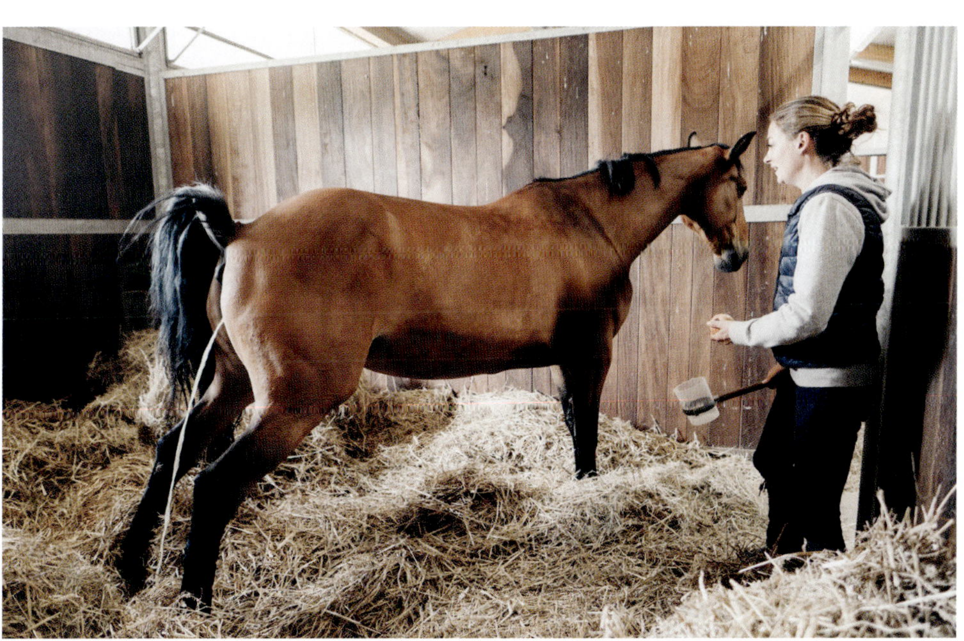

The first session: This mare is willing to urinate in the presence of a person who's standing still.

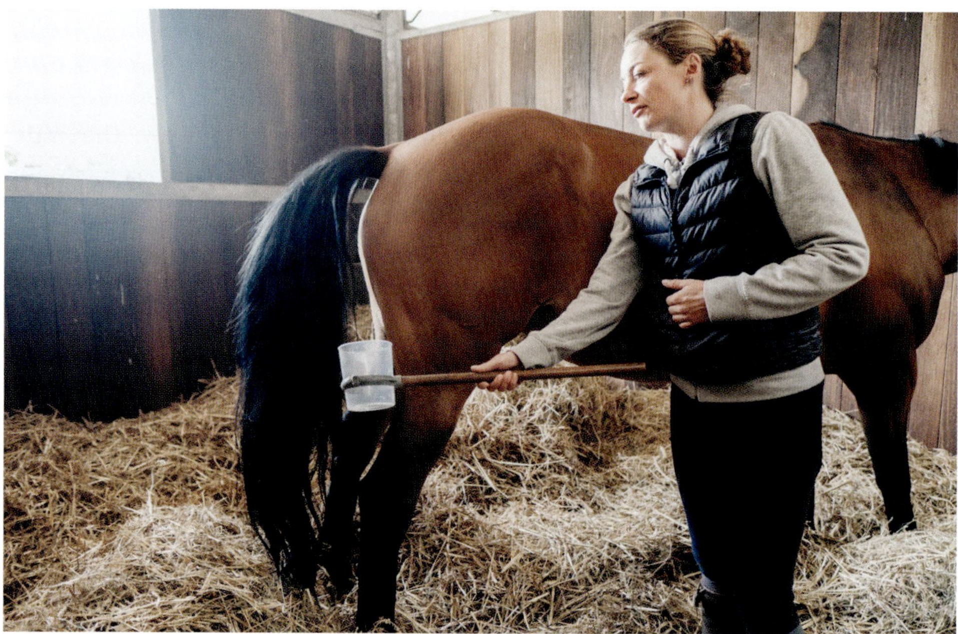

Fourth session: Without trying to actually collect the urine, the trainer confirms that she can move toward the horse's hindquarters with the container without the horse moving away.

looking for food as he follows you into his stall, and then he isn't thinking about urinating anymore. Stand in a neutral position, without putting your hands into your pockets or your treat bag.

1. As soon as the horse goes into a urination stance, click and approach to reward him.

2. It's likely that the horse will hold back at this point, trying to figure out what you're doing; wait, or even leave the stall.

3. When the horse returns to a urination stance, click and reward him.

4. Wait.

5. He shouldn't hold it for too much longer, and will start urinating.

6. Click, reward him, and repeat this several times during urination.

This first session might take some time—you'll have to wait around for the moment the horse is ready to urinate, and since your clicks and rewards are going to interrupt him you'll have to wait even more before he does it. Think of this time as an investment. You're not wasting it, because you'll gain it back every time you need to collect urine in the future and it's fast and easy, thanks to this training.

In the second session, follow the same steps the same way. You shouldn't have to wait as long as you did during the first session. In the third session, in the same setting:

1. As soon as the horse goes into a urination stance, click and approach him to reward him.

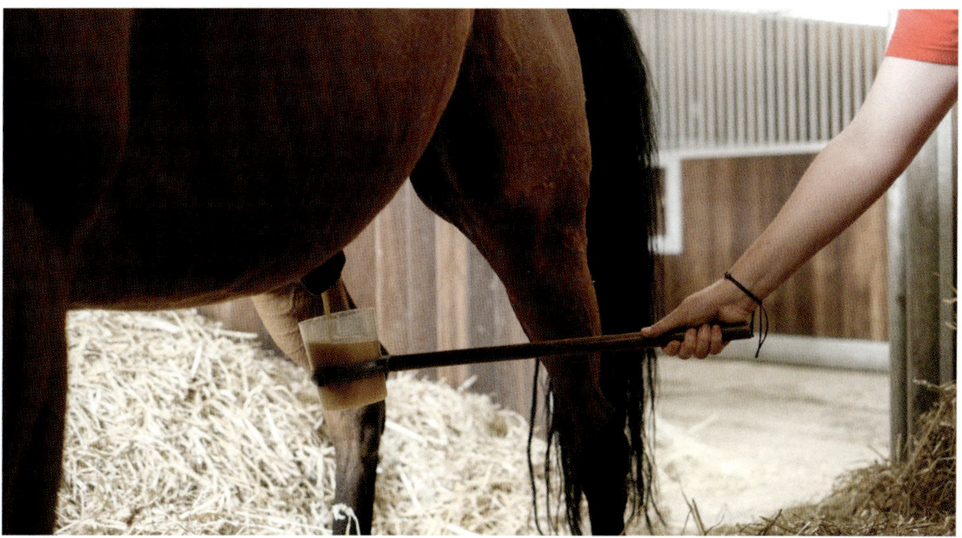

Fifth session, step 4: collecting the urine.

2. However many times he returns to this position after you interrupt him, click and reward him each time.

3. Click and reward once during urination.

4. Move toward the horse's hindquarters and hold out your arm for one second.

5. Click, bend your arm again, and return to the horse's head to reward him.

In the fourth session, in the same setting again:

1. As soon as the horse goes into a urination stance, click and approach him to reward him.

2. However many times he returns to this position after you interrupt him, click and reward him each time.

3. Click and reward him once during urination.

4. Move toward the horse's hindquarters and hold out your arm for three seconds.

5. Click, bend your arm again, and return to the horse's head to reward him.

For the fifth session, bring the container with you.

1. As soon as the horse goes into a urination stance, click and approach him to reward him.

2. However many times he returns to this position after you interrupt him, click and reward him each time.

3. Click and reward him once during urination.

4. Move toward the horse's hindquarters and hold out the container by its handle to collect some urine.

5. Click, move the container away from the horse, and return to his head to reward him.

For this exercise, there are multiple variations available to you. If you can tell your horse is very relaxed and completely comfortable being approached while he urinates, you can try to collect some urine in the third session instead of waiting until the fifth. For horses who are more worried about having you around, extending the process over five sessions should help put them at ease. If you notice the horse holding back when you move around, you'll need to add a few more sessions before you move your arm or the container toward the horse. If it's the container that's making the horse nervous, repeat the stage where you're holding out your arm with nothing in your hand a few more times, and plan on a session where you introduce the container to the horse and touch him with its handle, as in the Clipping exercise, using approach-retreat and rewards (see page 93).

On Demand

Once your horse is trained with this exercise, you can teach him a signal so he'll urinate on command. Obviously the horse has to be in a comfortable environment for this to work, and you can't ask him to urinate again if he just did it by himself. But it can still be surprisingly effective. When the horse urinates, give your signal, click, and reward him. Repeat this whenever you're working on this exercise and the horse starts to urinate. He may start trying to see whether you'll reward him for going into a urination stance even if he doesn't actually urinate; you might be fooled once or twice, but soon you'll learn to wait until you see some actual urine. Keep giving the signal in the same place at first, and eventually you'll be able to generalize it to other locations.

Common Mistakes

Refusing to reward the horse after clicking because the horse stopped urinating. He may have stopped because of the sound of the click—but if your click (or click of the tongue or other marker) was given while he *was* urinating, then he should get his reward.

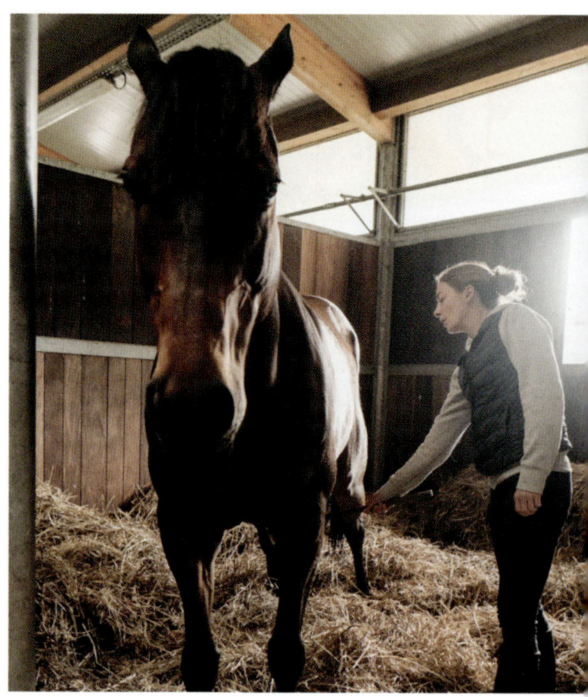

Provide the horse with a place he's going to want to urinate, such as a stall with plenty of fresh bedding.

 — **PREPARING YOUR HORSE OR DONKEY FOR VETERINARY CARE**

Stretching

What's the Point?

Stretching is good for the horse's body. Before or after a work session, or while in recovery—and it also yields potentially valuable diagnostic information. A veterinarian may use stretching to check the mobility of the horse's neck, for example. Some horses don't like to bend their neck, and training them to do it voluntarily when asked is helpful.

What You'll Need

- Food rewards.
- A bag to hold rewards.
- A close-range target.
- A long-range target (on the end of a pole or a stick).

What You Want the Horse to Do

Stay in contact with a target that changes position.

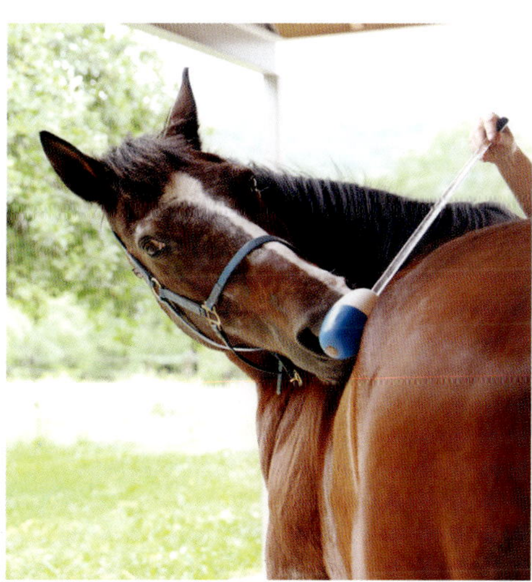

To ask the horse to hold this position, instead of clicking as soon as he touches the target, I wait a couple seconds.

✦ What You Do

For this exercise, I recommend the voluntary contact technique. Manipulating the horse's head and neck yourself is technically possible, but I think it's more valuable to ask the horse to perform the movement on his own, and see whether he's willing and able to hold specific positions. You could also do this by luring the horse with food so his nose follows your hand—this is a positive reinforcement technique called lure-reward. If you're working with an untrained horse, lure-reward works without any prior preparation; but you risk the horse getting worked up and trying to grab your fingers when he's going for the carrot. By contrast, if you ask him to follow a target with the promise of a future reward he can depend on, he'll be calm and relaxed, and he'll hold a position if you ask him to. If he can't stretch as far in a certain direction as you expect, you'll learn it without putting your fingers at risk.

✦ Step by Step: Raising and Lowering the Head with the Clicker and a Target

First, train your horse to be polite when you're holding treats with the Statue exercise (see page 38). You should also practice asking him to touch a target until he does it consistently. If you haven't reached these goals with him, review these exercises and work on them before you start this one (see page 34).

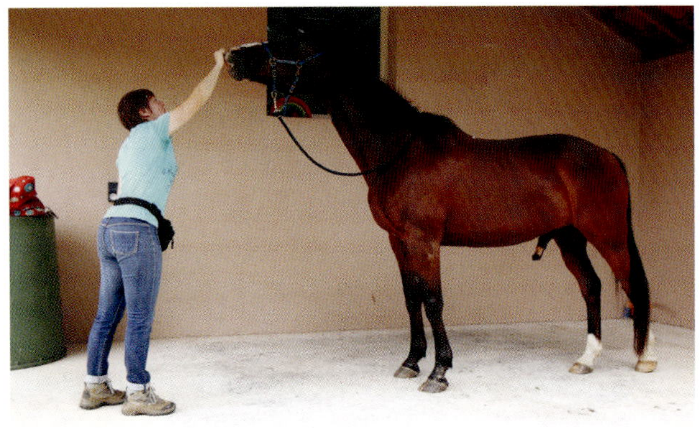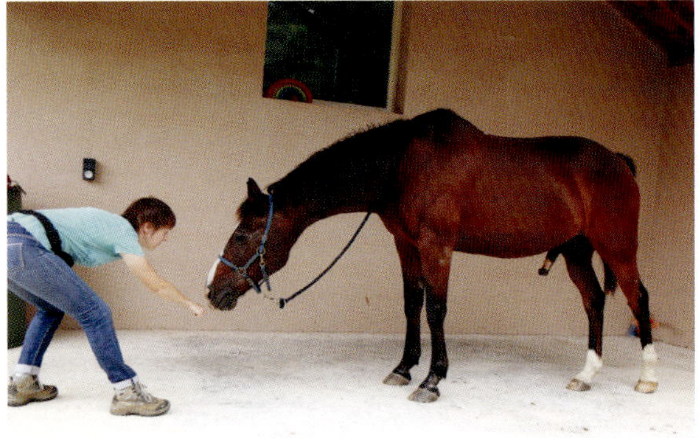

You can ask your horse to raise (left) or lower (right) his head with your hand as the target for him to touch.

Hold your close-range target in one hand and face the horse. Click and reward for each of these steps when your horse touches the target:

1. Hold the target in front of the horse, at his chest level, and wait for him to touch it.

2. Ask the horse to keep touching the target for at least three seconds.

3. Hold the target in front of the horse, at his knee level, far enough in front of him that he'll have to stretch both forward and down to reach it but not so far that he feels like he needs to take a step forward, and wait for him to touch it. (If he steps forward consistently, work on this step with him in his stall and a barrier like a rope across the doorway to prevent him from moving toward you).

4. Hold the target in front of the horse at the level of his eyes so he has to stretch upward to touch it.

5. Repeat each of these several times, and ask for contact for the duration your veterinarian or equine physical therapist has advised.

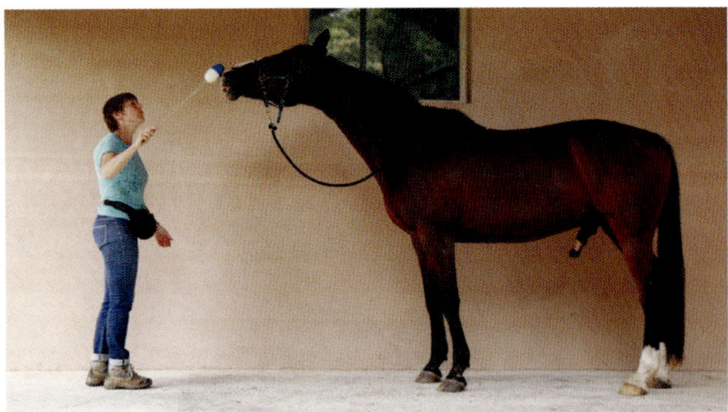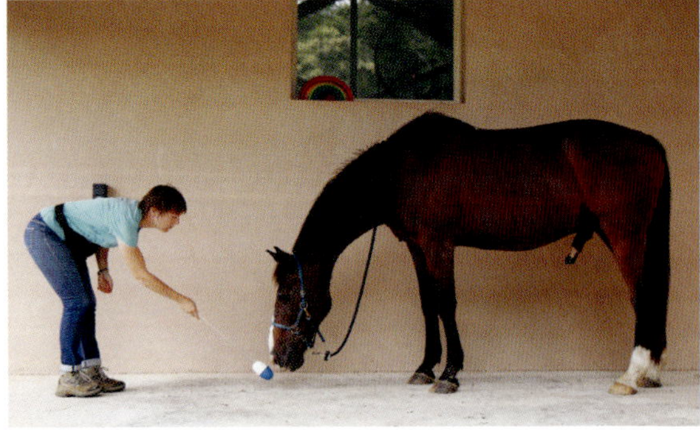

With a long-range target on the end of a pole or stick, you won't have to reach as far when you're asking the horse to stretch.

 — **PREPARING YOUR HORSE OR DONKEY FOR VETERINARY CARE**

The long-range target will help you ask your horse to stretch upward, especially if he's tall, and it'll save you from having to bend over as far when you ask him to stretch downward. A short-range target is still good to start with—and your closed fist can also work as a short-range target. I like to use a closed fist here to distinguish this exercise from the contact with a flat hand that I use when I'm working toward carrying out a treatment on the horse (as for Administering Eye Care on page 137). Horses usually find it easier to touch a target below their head height than a target above it. If your horse has trouble stretching upward, move your target upward more gradually.

◆ Step by Step: Stretching the Neck with the Clicker and a Target

1. Repeat these steps on both sides of the horse, clicking and rewarding each step:

2. Position yourself behind the horse's shoulder and offer him the target slightly behind his head.

3. Gradually move the target backward and downward, toward his shoulder level.

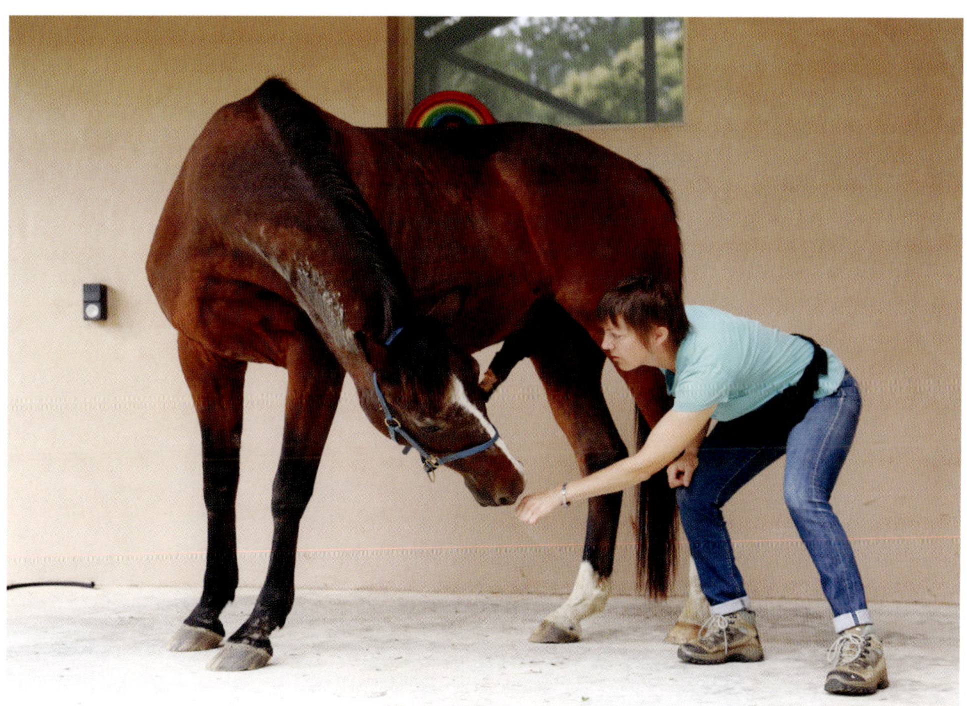

The horse doesn't get a click and a reward if he doesn't touch my fist. So he makes an effort to stretch more. If he really struggled with this movement or refused to try to touch my fist, I'd make sure to ask for less next time. The advantage of this clicker-and-target method is that we aren't physically forcing the horse into a position, and the horse knows a treat is coming but it isn't right in front of him tempting him to lunge for it.

Ask him to bend downward, as if he were scratching his hindquarters with his teeth.

Variation with a Long-Range Target

- Without changing sides, extend the pole of the long-range target over the horse's back to ask for flexion to the opposite side.

Be aware: for this to succeed, you must train your horse to accept objects passing from one side of him to the other over his back. If you haven't done this, he might be frightened by the sudden appearance of the long-range target on the side it wasn't on before—and if he moves away from it, he'll be moving into you, standing on his other side. Many horses are perfectly fine with this, but it pays to make sure your horse is one of them before you do this variation.

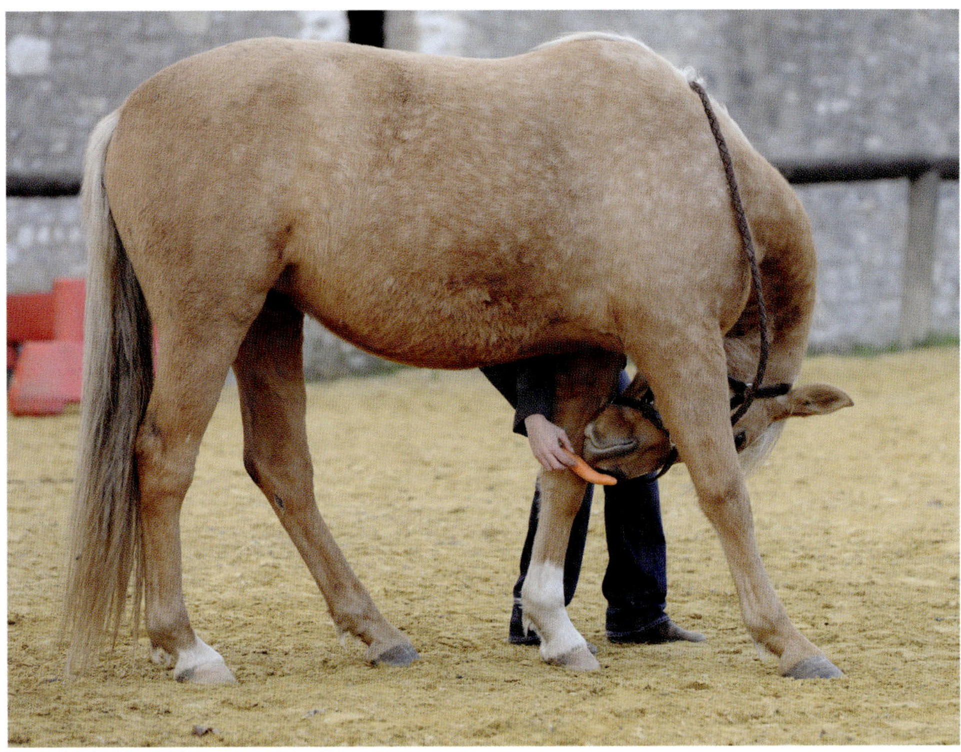

Luring the horse into a stretch with a carrot helps you check his mobility with minimal training, but he may get impatient and rush to grab for the food instead of holding the position you want. Using the clicker-and-target method is better.

 — **PREPARING YOUR HORSE OR DONKEY FOR VETERINARY CARE**

GLOSSARY

A change in behavior as the result of past experience is what ethology researchers call **learning**. There are different kinds of learning processes. Scientists have named some of them after work carried out in laboratories. Educators and trainers use techniques in practice that also have technical names. Here is a non-exhaustive list of some terms you might run into when you're learning more about how to train horses, ponies, and donkeys.

Habituation: A phenomenon which leads a previously existing response to diminish and disappear. An animal may initially react strongly to stimulation; then he learns to be indifferent to it, if there are no consequences that follow it. If you repeat a stimulus that is initially frightening—the noise of a clipper running, for example—without exceeding your horse's ability to tolerate it for short periods (he may still be afraid, but he's not afraid enough to run away), and you gradually move closer until you can touch him with the clipper without bothering him, you are making use of habituation.

Sensitization: The opposite of habituation. Upon repetition of a stimulus that doesn't initially elicit a response, the animal learns to react more and more strongly. When you're handling a horse, if you exceed his tolerance—for example, by bringing a clipper too close to him too quickly—you can create stronger avoidance responses in him, which is the opposite of what you wanted. This is the phenomenon that makes it so crucial to look for signs of fear or distress in the equine you're handling; but it's also the phenomenon that teaches a horse to be increasingly responsive to your requests, as he learns success earns him rewards and becomes sensitive to your signals.

Positive reinforcement: A phenomenon linked to what is called "operant conditioning," in which the animal, through trial and error, develops an interest in repeating behavior that earns him a reward. Typically this reward, also called a "reinforcer," is food.

The word "positive," in this context, refers to the addition of an element—the reward—after the desired behavior occurs. Clicker training is a technique based on positive reinforcement.

Negative reinforcement: A phenomenon linked to what is called "operant conditioning," in which the animal, through trial and error, develops an interest in repeating behavior that causes something unpleasant he is experiencing to go away. With a horse, the unpleasant experience is usually pressure (on the halter, against his sides, or against his mouth) that will stop when the horse does what we want him to do. The word "negative," in this context, refers to the subtraction of an element—the unpleasant experience—after the desired behavior occurs. Approach-retreat is a technique based on negative reinforcement. Horseback riding in general, in the European classical tradition, is based on the use of various kinds of negative reinforcement, too.

Reinforcements and punishments: In the field of learning theory, we also talk about punishment; in this technical context, "punishment" refers to anything that makes a behavior decrease in frequency or stop, while "reinforcement" refers to anything that makes a behavior increase in frequency. While you may be picturing a slap or a whipping in response to undesirable behavior when you read the word "punishment," in this context, an action only qualifies as punishment if it actually makes the undesirable behavior less likely—if it causes learning to occur. If an action only creates fear, without doing anything to alter behavior in a meaningful and systematic way, no learning occurs; the horse is afraid and in pain, and doesn't know why. He may be able to associate the treatment he receives with other things that allow him to predict that that treatment is coming—the place where it happens, the person who does it, the material around him when it happens, a noise that precedes it. But punishment can't be effective, in the context of learning, unless you think about it from the horse's point of view: is the action you intend to take going to help the horse understand which behavior you find undesirable, and which behavior you wanted instead? If the horse is engaging in undesirable behavior for a reason, is the action you intend to take going to address that reason, or not?

In learning theory, any reinforcement method is in a sense also punishment, whether the reinforcement is positive or negative: increasing the frequency of one behavior means decreasing the frequency of another. If you train a horse to respond to your requests correctly, then you've succeeded in eliminating behavior that would be an incorrect response to your request. As the terms are used in this context, if your horse halts in response to a vocal cue, that means you've reinforced halting and punished moving forward or backward. It can be difficult to use this vocabulary this way—to think that technically, you're punishing your horse when you reward him, if the reward decreases the frequency of an incorrect response! But digging deeper into learning theory means picking up its vocabulary, even when that vocabulary means something different outside a scientific context.

Desensitization: This term encompasses multiple techniques, and did not originate with scientists studying learning. It is now used in the field of learning theory to describe gradual exposure to a stimulus that could be frightening, without ever reaching a point where an animal starts to show fear responses. The "approach and retreat" technique, which involves exposing an animal to a potentially frightening stimulus and then removing it when the animal stays still and tolerates it, is a type of operant conditioning that fits into this category: the animal learns that if he keeps moving, the sound of a clipper running, for example, will continue, but it will stop if he stands still—negative reinforcement. The volume has to start out low enough that the animal is willing to try standing still near it, and you have to shut the sound off when he does try it. If you simply leave the sound playing continuously, that's **immersion**. And in that case, an eventual lack of reaction to the sound by the animal doesn't mean he's learned anything; it may just be resignation. No matter what he does, the sound won't stop, so he's given up on searching for a solution. The line between conditioning and immersion is defined by the amount of the potentially frightening stimulus and your responsiveness to signs of fear or relaxation in the animal—it's thin, but crucial.

Approach-retreat: This technique involves gradually approaching an animal—in this book, a horse or another equine—with equipment, a noise, or a part of your body, until he no longer responds to it with fear. Each step in the "approach" stops as soon as the horse stands still; if he moves, the stimulus continues, but at a lower intensity (farther away from him or less loudly, depending on the stimulus). This is a learning process based on negative reinforcement: an unpleasant element of the horse's experience goes away if he does what you want him to do. It can be combined with positive reinforcement by also giving the horse a reward for standing still. This is what I recommend for the Clipping exercise (see page 93).

Clicker training: This term covers a set of techniques that all use positive reinforcement. The key is to teach the animal a signal—most often the characteristic click of a clicker—that the trainer can use when the animal performs the behavior the trainer is seeking. Then, within the next few seconds, the trainer rewards the animal. Techniques for encouraging the animal to try the right behavior (since he has to perform it before you can click and reward him to tell him it was correct) will vary. In this book, I commonly explain how to use touching a target to guide a horse toward the correct behavior. The trainer should also choose an environment that makes it easy for the animal to perform the right behavior. It's possible to "capture" a behavior the animal does naturally by waiting for it to occur and then using the clicker (as in the Collecting Urine Samples exercise on page 160).

Lure-reward: Luring involves attracting an animal with food. He's following the food, not any instructions or signals, and by doing so, he is guided through the correct behavior. This is different from the rewards given in clicker training; there, rewards do not appear until the correct behavior has already been offered. Luring tends to take up some of the animal's attention, which means he doesn't always form an association between his behavior and obtaining the food—he doesn't learn anything. However, luring can sometimes help you elicit a behavior enough times in a row that you can begin involving a signal in the process; you should remove the lure and continue using the signal to request the behavior going forward.

Target: An object that serves as a goal; an animal can be trained to maintain contact with a target, or learn not to be afraid by touching a target that is the object of his fear. Your hand can be a target, too. Targets are commonly used in clicker training, as you can see in multiple exercises in this book.

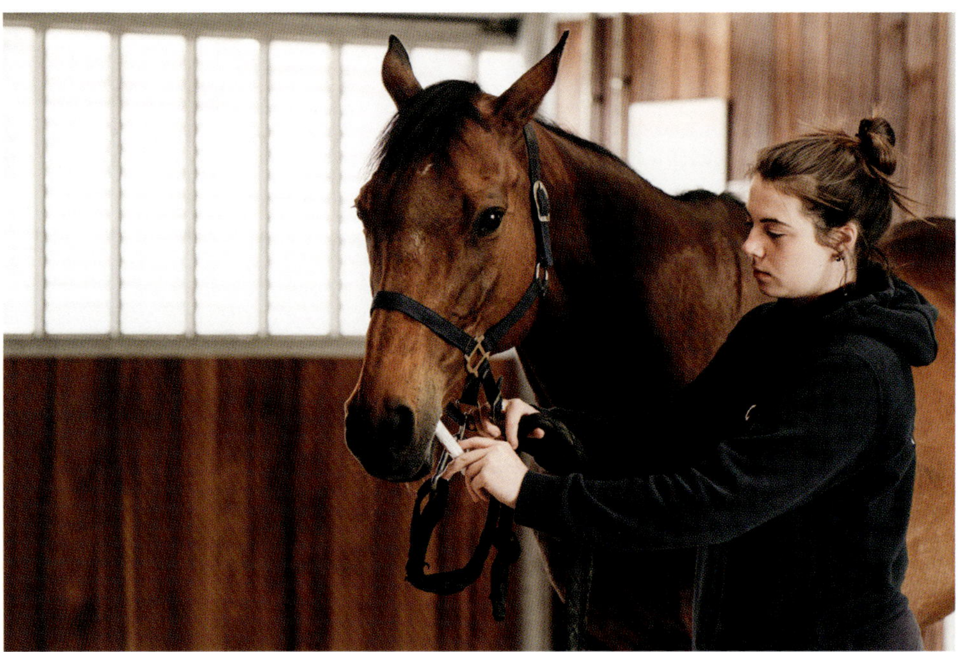

You can combine multiple techniques to help your horse understand how to cooperate. Overall, positive reinforcement—clicker training—creates good experiences for him and counteracts the unpleasant experience of undergoing veterinary care.

SUMMARY TABLE

	Progressive Habituation	Approach-retreat	Approach-retreat + clicker training	Clicker training with a target (object or hand) /voluntary contact	Clicker training + "stop button"
Touching Sensitive Places		X	X		X
Touching the Gums			X		
Taking the Temperature		X	X		X
Clipping	X	X	X		X
Bathtime		X	X		X
Applying a Spray	X	X	X		X
Preparing for Dental Care	X	X	X	X	
Using an Inhaler or Nebulizer	X	X	X	X	
Performing an Injection or a Blood Test		X	X		X
Deworming or Administering Medication Orally		X	X	X	X
Administering Eye Care			X	X	X
Positioning a Limb		X	X	X	
Weighing with a Scale		X	X	X	
Guiding a Horse into a Treatment Room	X		X		
Collecting Urine Samples			X		
Stretching				X	

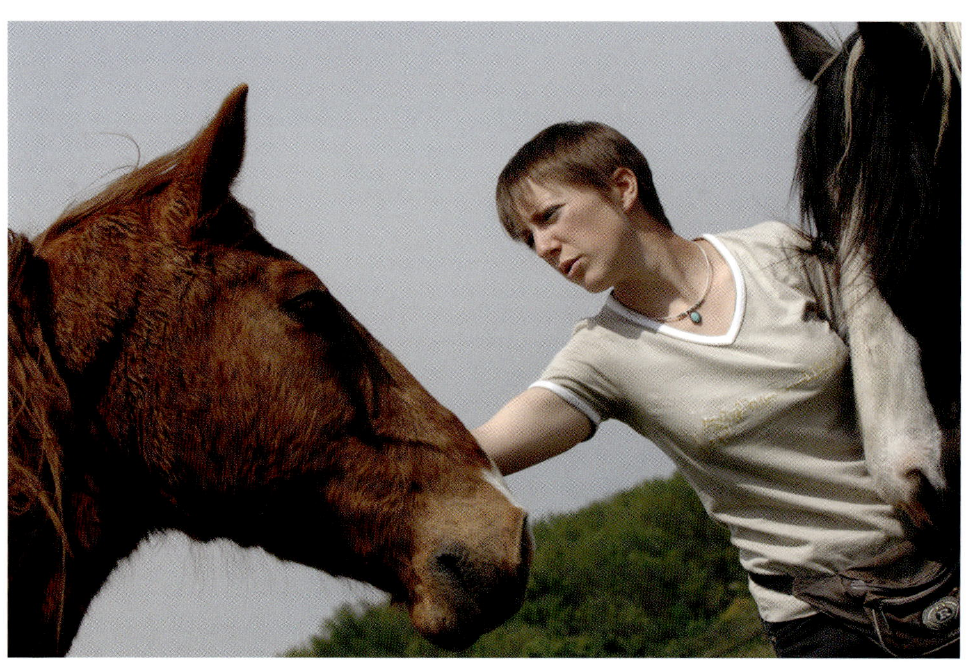

A special thank-you to horses like Sanson, who are our best teachers, and who help us teach our fellow humans more effectively, too.

ACKNOWLEDGMENTS

Thank you to equine veterinarians Julie Dauvillier, Sophie Mercier, Vincent Boureau and Tristan Deguillaume for their careful proofreading of the French edition and their wise comments, as well as Claire Scicluna for motivating me to address this topic in the first place.

Thank you to Alice de Boyer des Roches, doctor of ethology, for her support, her careful proofreading of the French edition, and her commitment to the well-being of horses.

Thank you to the French National Horse Racing Federation, and in particular Dr. Hélène Bourguignon, for the trust she has placed in me and the interest she has in the well-being of racehorses and all others.

I would also like to thank the French National Horse Racing Federation's technical team for their welcome, and I would like to emphasize the quality of their relationships with their horses: Louise L'Hermitte, Mickael Megissier, Anaïs Sauvage, and Léa Fortin.

Thank you to the Vallon stable for hosting us during photo sessions.

Thank you to Dr. Agnès Debarre and Dr. Élodie Danjou for taking part in the photoshoots used to illustrate this book, and for their kindness during consultations. I also need to thank the Swiss national stud farm, which made it possible to include the photographs of the mares on the scales.

Thank you to photographers Marie Roig-Pons, Jérémy Durand, Alice de Boyer des Roches, Eva Garnerone and Ludovic Fournet for their time and the quality of their work; and I can't leave out the pre-existing photographs taken by Alain Laurioux and Isabelle Arnon.

Thank you to Aude, Théophile, and Ariane, who followed the instructions to set up for photographs when I was behind the lens.

Thank you to Laurie, Claire, Isabelle, Isabelle, and Thomas, who also took part in the sessions in front of the lens with Marie and Alice; and Maëlle, Françoise, Corinne, and Évelyne, for the sessions with Alain.

Thank you to Véronique de Saint Vaulry on one side of the lens, and Coline, Jean-Philippe, and Jim on the other; and to Véronique a second time for her drawings and her attentive proofreading of the French edition.

Thank you to Anne Pasquet and the Ânes Victoires association for photographs of long ears, with the participation of Victoire, Damien, Georgina, and Danie.

Thank you to the owners and horses who trusted me to help them with complicated treatments. I'm thinking in particular of Pollux, Lockerby, and Big Red for eye care; Lorcan for a dressing for a hind hoof; Sanson, for everything from dewormer to injections including eye care; Señorita, for contact with sensitive places; and all the others I'm undoubtedly forgetting …
Thank you to the horses Kako, Luciole, Victor, and Jack, who are on the front lines of my daily experiments.

Thank you to Déesse, Diana, Pink Pearl, Tardif, Danover, Dutch Dream, Éclat, Maharo, Yesterday Cat, Nélimère, Réhézite, Savane, Qualoubet, Bribone, Coléa, Olana, Quyrus, Zelamar, Alakhia, Dalida, Vivi, Meknès, Inespérée, and Petit Nîmois, for their work as models.

Thank you to the donkeys Mica, Galice, Anaba, Gribouille, Good, and Pépita.

REFERENCES

1. Desbrosse F., 2007. "Restraint techniques," [Les techniques de contention], *Proceedings of the 35th AVEF Conference*, National Center in Deauville, p. 218–233.
2. Pearson G., Reardon R., Keen J. & Waran, N., 2020. "Difficult Horses: Prevalence, Approaches to Management of, and Understanding of How they Develop by Equine Veterinarians," *Equine Veterinary Education*, doi.org/10.1111/eve.13354
3. Hinde R., 1979. *Towards Understanding Relationships*, Academic Press, London.
4. Hausberger M., Roche H., Henry S. & Visser K., 2008. "A review of the human-horse relationship," *Applied Animal Behaviour Science*, 109, p. 1–24.
5. Link to the YouTube video under the title "Tiger træning / Copenhagen Zoo": https://www.youtube.com/watch?v=yDGEuihopWs (last visited 1/31/2021)
6. Pryor K., 2009. *Reaching the Animal Mind*, Scribner, New York.
7. *Ibid.*
8. Ramirez K., 2012. *How to Become a Top Trainer?* Conference in Munich. April 20–22, 2012.
9. Personal observation of professionals who teach training techniques with certain species for example, dogs and consulted me to transfer their approaches to horses, or marine mammal caretakers who exclusively apply positive reinforcement on these animals but have used dog trainers who base their work on negative reinforcement to train their dogs, when they have the theoretical knowledge to mix their training tools.
10. "ISES: 10 training principles," from https://equitationscience.com/learning-theory/ (accessed 01/02/2021); translated and adapted for ease of use. You will find the exhaustive version written by ISES and the educational poster at the indicated URL.
11. Roche H., 2020. *Apprendre à observer les chevaux: Dans les pas des scientifiques* [Learning to observe horses: In the footsteps of scientists], Éditions Delachaux & Niestlé.

12. Gleerup K.B. & Lindergaard C., 2016. "Recognition and Quantification of Pain in the Horse: A Tutorial Review." *Equine Veterinary Education*, 28, p. 47–57.

13. Dalla Costa E., Minero M., Lebelt D., Stucke D., Canali E. & Leach M., 2014. "Development of the Horse Grimace Scale (HGS) as a Pain Assessment Tool in Horses Undergoing Routine Castration," PloSONE, doi.org/10.1371/journal.pone.0092281

14. Dalla Costa E., Stucke D., Dai F., Minero M., Leach M. & Lebelt D., 2016. "Using the Horse Grimace Scale (HGS) to Assess Pain Associated to Acute Laminitis in Horses (*Equus caballus*)," *Animals*, Aug 3;6(8):47. doi: 10.3390/ani6080047

15. Coneglian M.M., Borges T.D., Weber S.H., Bertagnon H.G. & Michelotto P.V., 2020. "Use of the Horse Grimace Scale to Identify and Quantify Pain Due to Dental Disorders in Horses." *Applied Animal Behaviour Science*, 104970.

16. Gleerup K., Forkman B., Lindegaard C. & Andersen P., 2015. "An Equine Pain Face," *Veterinary Anaesthesia and Analgesia*, 42, p. 103–114.

17. Merkies K., Ready C., Frakas L. & Hodder A., 2019. "Eye Blink Rates and Eyelid Twitches as a NonInvasive Measure of Stress in the Domestic Horse," *Animals*, 9, 562, doi:10.3390/ani9080562

18. Gleerup *et al.*, 2015. *Op. cit.*

19. Bussières G., Jacques C., Lainay O., Beauchamp G., Leblond A., Cadoré J.L., Desmaizières M., Cuvelliez S.G. & Troncy E., 2008. "Development of a Composite Orthopaedic Pain Scale in Horses." *Research in Veterinary Science*, 85 (2), p. 294–306.

20. Van Dierendonck M., Burden F., Rickards K., van Loon J., 2020. "Monitoring Acute Pain in Donkeys with the Equine Utrecht University Scale for Donkeys Composite Pain Assessment (EQUUSDONKEYCOMPASS) and the Equine Utrecht University Scale for Donkey Facial Assessment of Pain (EQUUSDONKEYFAP)," *Animals*, 10, 354 doi:10.3390/ani10020354

21. Burden F. & Thiemann A., 2015. "Donkeys Are Different." *Journal of Equine Veterinary Science*, 35, p.376–382.

22. *Ibid.*

23. *Ibid*; Orth E., Gonzalez F., Pastrana C., Berger J., Le Jeune S., Davis E. & McLean A., 2020. "Development of a Donkey Grimace Scale to Recognize Pain in Donkeys (*Equus donkey*) Post Castration," *Animals* 10, 1411; doi:10.3390/ani10081411.

24. Orth *et al.*, 2020. *Op. cit.*

25. Van Dierendonck *et al.*, 2020. *Op. cit.*

26. *Ibid.*

27. Haines A. & Goliszek J., 2019. "Donkey and Mule Behaviour for the Veterinary Team," *Equine*, 3/1, p. 27–32.

28. *Ibid.*

29. I*bid* and personal observations of scratching, movement, and switching of the tail.

30. Burden F. & Thiemann A., 2015. *Op. cit.*

31. Le Moal C., Mespoulhès-Rivière C., Diederich C., Wiggers L., Robert C., Grimard B., Gilbert C., 2016. "Bien-être du cheval hospitalisé en clinique vétérinaire: évaluation et impact de l'enrichissement environnemental" [Well-being of the horse hospitalized in a veterinary clinic: evaluation and impact of environmental enrichment]. 42nd Equine Research Day, Paris, March 17, 2016, p. 165–167.

32. Lansade L., Neveux C., Valenchon M., Moussu C., Yvon J.M., Pasquier F. & Lévy F., 2011. "Enrichir l'environnement des chevaux permet d'améliorer leur bien-être, de diminuer leur émotivité et d'augmenter la sécurité des manipulateurs" [Enriching horses' environments helps improve their well-being, reduce their reactivity, and improve the safety of their handlers]. 37th Equine Research Day, Le Pin au Haras, February 24, 2011, p. 33–41.

33. De Boyer des Roches A., Peyrecave-Capo X., Rocafort-Ferrer G., Thomas A., Roche H., Desjardins I., Mounier L. & Cadoré J.L., 2020. "Welfare and Management of Decreased Visual Capacities and Pain in a Pony Suffering from Equine Recurrent Uveitis: A Clinical Case." *Equine Veterinary Education*, doi: 10.1111/eve.13365

34. I*bid*.

35. Ear twisting is specifically mentioned among the list of aversive practices to avoid in the second of the ten ISES principles at https://equitation-science.com/learningtheory/ (accessed 02/01/2021)

36. Sankey C., Henry S., Gorecka-Bruzda A., Richard-Yris M.-A. & Hausberger M., 2011. "Aliment ou grattage: quelle récompense pour le cheval?" [Food or scratching: which reward for the horse?] Report from 37th Equine Research Day.

37. Kiley-Worthington M., 1976. "The tail movement of Ungulates, Canids and Felids with particular reference to their causation and function as displays." *Behavior*, 56, p. 69–115; Waring G.H., 2003. *Horse Behavior.* New York: Noyes Publications.

38. McDonnell S., 2003. A *practical field guide to horse behavior—The Equid Ethogram.* Editions A division of the Bloodhorse, Inc., 375 pages.

39. Fureix C., Sankey C., Vallet A.S., André N. & Hausberger M., 2011. "Loin des yeux, loin du cœur! Les chevaux sont-ils sensibles à l'état attentionnel de l'homme lors d'une interaction?" [Out of sight, out of mind! Are horses sensitive to the direction of human attention during an interaction?] Report at the 37th Equine Research Day; Proops L. & McComb K., 2010. "Attributing

Attention: The Use of Human-Given Cues by Domestic Horses (*Equus caballus*)," *Animal Cognition*, 13, p.197–205.

40. Desbrosse F., 2007. O*p. cit.*

41. I*bid.*

42. I*bid.*

43. Feh C., 2005. "Relationships and communication in socially natural horse herds," in T*he Domestic Horse: The Evolution, Development and Management of its Behaviour*, edited by Daniel Mills and Sur McDonnell, Cambridge University Press.

44. Personal observations.

45. Pasquet H., 2004. L*es accidents et dommages corporels vétérinaires équins dans l'exercice de leur profession* [Accidents and injuries for equine veterinarians in the course of their jobs]. Veterinary doctoral thesis, Créteil.

46. Giniaux D., 2003. *Soulagez votre cheval aux doigts (et à l'œil!)* [Soothe your horse with your fingers (and eyes!)], Optipress, p. 87.

47. Desbrosses F., 2007. O*p. cit.*

48. Flakoll B., Ali A. & Saab C., 2017. "Twitching in veterinary procedures: How does this technique subdue horses?" *Journal of Veterinary Behavior*, 18, p. 23–28.

49. Personal observations and numerous testimonies.

50. Desbrosse F., 2007. O*p. cit.*

51. I*bid.*

52. Lansade L., Pichard G. & Leconte M., 2008. "Sensory Sensitivities: Components of a Horse's Temperament Dimension," A*pplied Animal Behaviour Science*, 114, p. 534–553.

53. Desbrosse F., 2007. O*p. cit.*, p. 218 and 220.

54. I*bid*, p. 220.

55. Example with description in the video "On Your Mark, Get Set, Start Button," https://video.clickertraining.com/programs/onyourmarkgetset-startbutton (consulted 9/19/2022).

56. P. Jardat, L. Calandreau, V. Ferreira, C. Gouyet, C. Parias, F. Reignier & L. Lansade. "Pet Directed Speech Improves Horses' Attention Toward Humans." *Scientific Reports*, 12, 4297, doi.org/10.1038/s4159802208109z

57. This effect has been studied in casino patrons, for example in Talmi et al., 2008. Human Pavlovian-Instrumental Transfer," T*he Journal of Neuroscience*, 28 (2), p. 360–368.

58. Gough M.R., 1999. "A note on the use of behavioural modification to aid clipping ponies." A*pplied Animal Behaviour Science*, 63, p. 171–175.

59. Pearson G., https://www.youtube.com/watch?v=OjoaUeZO5CA (accessed 1/17/2022).

60. Greiveldinger L., Veissier I. & Boissy A., 2007. "Emotional experience in sheep: predictability of a sudden event lowers subsequent emotional responses." *Physiology and Behavior*, 92: p. 675–683.

61. Couetil L. et al., 2020. "Equine Asthma: Current Understanding and Future Directions." *Frontiers in Veterinary Science*, doi.org/10.3389/fvets.2020.00450

62. Greiveldinger *et al. Op. cit.*

63. McDonnell S., 2000. "How to rehabilitate horses with injection shyness (or any procedure noncompliance)." Proceedings of the annual convention of the AAEP, 2000, 46, p. 168–172.

64. Ramirez K., 1999. *Animal Training: Successful Animal Management Through Positive Reinforcement*. Shed Aquarium, Chicago, p. 141.

65. De Boyer des Roches *et al. Op. cit.*

66. *Ibid.*

67. Video of the pony Rocky at age 14 (in 2018): https://www.youtube.com/watch?v=gsCOS3IAttU

68. https://equipedia.ifce.fr/elevageetentretien/alimentation/nutritionetration/estimationdupoids (accessed 1/27/2021)

69. Fureix *et al.*; Proops & McComb. *Op. cit.*

70. De Saint Vaulry V., 2005. *Quand le cheval a peur* [When the Horse Is Afraid], Éditions Vigot, p. 273–274.

INDEX

Page numbers in *italics* indicate illustrations.

 — **PREPARING YOUR HORSE OR DONKEY FOR VETERINARY CARE**